From Both En
Stethosc

Getting through breast cancer - by a doctor who knows

by Dr Kathleen Thompson

From Both Ends Of The Stethoscope
Getting through breast cancer – by a doctor who knows

© Kathleen Thompson

Published by Faito Books
First published 2015

The rights of Kathleen Thompson to be identified as the author of this work have been asserted in accordance with the Copyright, Designs and Patents Act 1988.

British Library Cataloguing in Publication data available

Paperback ISBN ------978-0-9935083-0-1
Ebook ISBN-----------978-0-9935083-1-8

www.faitobooks.co.uk

Book cover design by J and C Heath
Typesetting by E Hayward

Everything described in this book really happened, and has been recreated from memory as truly as possible. However, names, identifying characteristics (sometimes even gender), dialogue and details of the people and institutions involved have been changed to protect privacy. Some minor characters have been merged and if any name resembles that of an actual person, this is purely coincidental.

While the author has made every effort to ensure that the information in this book was correct at time of press, she does not assume and hereby disclaims any liability to any party for any loss, damage, or disruption caused by errors or omissions, whether such errors or omissions result from negligence, accident, or any other cause.

The information provided in this book originates from many sources. These are not always specifically referenced for each statement, however the main sources are included in the further information sections at the end of each chapter.

For the most important people in my life, my children,
and, of course, their spouses.

Thanks to my wonderful family and friends who provided so
much love and support whilst I went through my treatment and
afterwards, and to my good friend Margaret Graham for her mentoring
and guidance throughout this book.

A message to the reader

I am a UK doctor — used to treating patients, not being one — but one day my world turned upside-down, and like Alice, I found myself falling and spinning down a long rabbit hole. I tumbled out at the wrong end of my stethoscope, where I was told I had breast cancer.

In this book, I describe what having breast cancer is like, the treatment process, and how to get the best care. I also explain why we get cancer, what we can do to reverse this and how to make sense of what we may read on the internet.

During my treatment I learned that the NHS has good features and many dedicated staff. Overall, my care was outstanding, and I am deeply grateful to the doctors, nurses and other staff who cared for me.

As with all things, occasionally mistakes were made. This does not reflect on the competence of the individuals involved – I don't believe any of them were incompetent. I discuss the errors as well as the excellent care. Both were a significant part of my cancer experience and will, I hope, help patients and their relatives and friends to navigate their way through the system. I hope they may also help health care workers in their important work.

This book is intended only to provide an insight and general guidance on breast cancer — it is not a textbook, and it certainly should not be used in place of seeking medical help. Everyone is different, and everyone's cancer is different. It is very important to consult a doctor as soon as you think you may have a problem, and to keep seeing doctors throughout your illness.

Prologue

However did this happen to me?

The nurse asked me to lie on the couch by the ultrasound machine.
'The doctor will be here soon.'
A tall man with white hair walked through the door and smiled. He sat down next to the machine.
Looking straight into my eyes, he spoke. 'The problem is, we've seen a lump on your mammogram. So I need to look at it with this ultrasound.'
Very gently, he pulled down my blue gown and exposed my breasts. I flinched as he squirted a blob of cold gel onto my skin. He pressed the ultrasound probe onto the blob, and moved it slowly over my right breast for a few minutes. He pointed to the fuzzy image on the small screen.
'This is the lump — it's about 2cm wide.' His voice was quiet but firm. 'Do you see the irregular shape, and these little bright flecks? These are worrying.'
He looked at me as he said this. His blue eyes offered sympathy and strength.
The screen looked like an ancient TV with a lousy reception. I couldn't make out any lump—but I understood 'irregular shape' and 'worrying' well enough.
'I see you're a doctor. Where do you practice?' he continued.
'I was a paediatrician, but now I work in drug research.'
'Oh? Interesting.' His smile morphed into a serious expression, 'I need to take a biopsy of this lump. We have these neat little things now.' He held a small black box between his finger and thumb.
'I'm going to press this box over the lump, then push this button, and a needle will shoot out and take the sample. It'll make a loud click, but it won't hurt, because I'm going to numb you first.'
I lay on the couch in the semi-darkness, watching him fill a small syringe with local anaesthetic. The cold wall, pressing against my left arm, forced me to concentrate. Everything was unreal — surreal. What was I doing here? I'd only come in for a check. My left hand gripped the coarse material of the hospital gown as if it was a survival rope. My right hand was visible to him and the nurse, so I forced it to relax.

Lifting the small syringe towards me, he injected the anaesthetic into my breast. It stung, but I hid the pain with a smile. 'No, it doesn't hurt. It's fine. It's a lovely day outside. I don't expect you'll have much chance to enjoy it, stuck in here.'

Somehow I controlled my voice — but tears were streaming down my face. I hoped the darkened room would hide them.

Then, a loud click shattered the quiet. He'd taken the biopsy, and he was right, it hadn't hurt.

'Well done. All finished. Nurse will pop a dressing on for you. Then she'll take you to see the breast surgeon. Good luck with your research work.' And he was gone.

On an otherwise unremarkable spring day, my life had just changed forever.

Contents

Chapter 1

Introduction

Let's face it, cancer is what happens to other people. Poor souls, with the sword of Damocles swinging on a fraying thread over their heads, these are people who are inevitably going to die, and soon. Of course we feel sorry for them — we'll send them a card, a basket of fruit, some flowers, but we certainly don't have plans to join their exclusive club.

Well guess what? All of us have cancer cells in our bodies on a fairly regular basis, and more than one in three of us in the western world will experience some form of cancer during our lives. So I'm afraid there's a fairly high chance of 'us' becoming 'them'. Maybe you're reading this because you've already joined the 'club'.

The good news is, our bodies are very capable of fighting cancer. Indeed, most of the time cancer cells are destroyed as soon as they develop, much in the way that our immune system hunts down and destroys bacteria or viruses. Other times, the cancer sneaks through our defences, but even if it does, it can still be overcome. I say 'can' because despite all efforts, some people do succumb. To keep things in perspective though, many cancer sufferers live to a very respectable old age, and eventually fill up completely different columns in the 'cause of death' statistics.

Cancer is on the increase, and there are many theories as to why. So, what steps can we take to reduce our chance of getting cancer, or to help fight an existing cancer? I have some ideas for you inside this book.

But first, who am I? What qualifications do I have that would permit me to offer you advice in what could be an extremely traumatic time? I'm a medical doctor. I'm on the wrong side of fifty and divorced. I have two fabulous

1

children, a loving extended family and some good friends. I'd always worked hard, but I was starting to ease off, take up more hobbies and enjoy myself — when my life changed.

Like you, I never thought I would get cancer.

As a doctor, I would sympathise with cancer patients and offer them encouragement from within my armour-plated white-coat.

They were the patients, I was the doctor. Simple.

Even when my developing cancer crept into my consciousness, I ignored it, and my own advice.

Maybe it would just go away.

But it didn't, and I had to face the realisation that my life might be cut very short. Then, on top of that, I had to negotiate my way through complicated highly-specialised medical treatments and, on occasions, challenge medical decisions. I found this extremely hard, even as a doctor, because I was also a vulnerable patient, and I was depending on other doctors for my survival.

Cancer taught me a great deal. Primarily it taught me that diagnosis is not a death sentence. People can and do survive cancer, most of the time. However, being forced to face the possibility of my imminent demise, I gradually learned not to fear death either. I also learned to appreciate every day of this wonderful thing called life.

I have a lot to share with you, so welcome to Cancer Club —whether you have cancer yourself or you know someone who has.

Most of this book deals with breast cancer, but much of the information and advice within these pages can be applied to other cancers, especially as regards lifestyle and cancer risk. The majority of the information relates to the UK, and medical practice elsewhere may be different.

Summary:

Cancer cells appear in our bodies regularly, but most of the time our immune system destroys them. Sometimes cancer breaks through despite this. There are things we can do to help ourselves. Many people, although not all, can expect a complete cure from cancer.

Further Reading:

Cancer Research UK   http://goo.gl/9DsU0t

An updated list of all web addresses included in this book can be found at http://www.faitobooks.co.uk/links

Chapter 2

What is breast cancer? What is cancer, come to that?

Cancer means that some of our cells start to look and act abnormally. As the cells' appearance becomes more abnormal, so does their behaviour.

You may not think of cells having behaviour. Well, we're not talking about being rowdy in the classroom, or refusing to do the washing up — although in some ways cancer cells can actually be compared to unruly teenagers. Normally, cells grow to a certain size and then stop. Some cells have the ability to divide into two — others don't. The difference with cancer cells is that they ignore the body's instructions to stop growing and to stop dividing. So two cells become four cells, which become eight cells, and before you know it they have become millions.

As the tumour gets bigger, it seems to grow faster. Imagine a tumour the size of a pea — doubling means it would grow to the size of two peas. Still pretty insignificant? But when it has grown to the size of an egg, it will still only take the same time to double and reach the size of two eggs, and when it reaches the size of an orange, it will double just as quickly to the size of two oranges.

Cancer is like a parasite, it steals its nourishment from the body's normal cells, and the bigger it is, the more nourishment it steals. Once we reach two oranges worth of cancer cells, our bodies have a real struggle on their hands.

Normal cells have a respect for boundaries. They stay where they're supposed to be. Cancer cells invade other parts of the body. They may just spread nearby, but they can also spread into blood vessels or lymphatic vessels, which act like a railway system transporting the cancer cells to other parts of the body, such as the lungs or the liver. Once in the new area, they continue to divide and multiply, all the while choking the normal cells which are trying to do their work.

Why do cancer cells form at all?

Every now and then our body produces a dud cell — a reject. We have excellent internal surveillance systems, and our immune system usually spots and destroys these reject cells. But every now and then one slips through the net and starts growing and doubling, out of control.

So cancer cells are actually something we all live with a lot of the time. After someone has had cancer, the first thing they, and everyone else, want to know is — is it cured? Has the cancer gone? Have they beaten cancer?

But as our bodies frequently produce cancer cells, talking about being totally cancer-free is not meaningful. The equivalent would be asking whether we will remain free from any infection for the rest of our lives if we'd just recovered from pneumonia. The answer is an obvious no, because our bodies are exposed to infection all the time. We could get a cold next week, or we could even get pneumonia again. Getting hung up on being cured of cancer is natural, but a better idea is to accept that our body is frequently dealing with cancer cells, and in order for us to remain well we have to be able to keep destroying them as soon as they appear. How we can help our bodies do this is discussed in the course of this book.

What about breast cancer? Since 1997, it has grown to be the commonest cancer in the UK. So many will have been touched by it, either directly or indirectly.

Breast cancer is any cancer originating from breast cells.

The breast consists of different cells, and the commonest type of cancer is ductal cancer — from the cells lining the milk ducts. Lobular cancer is less common and is formed from cells of the lobules, which are small cavities into which the milk is secreted, before it travels along the milk ducts. Another term you may hear is DCIS (ductal carcinoma-in-situ). This also relates to the duct cells, but in this case the cells have become slightly abnormal and have not yet developed into full-blown cancer.

Because men also have small amounts of breast tissue, 1% of breast cancers occur in men. It's important to remember that they also need a great deal of emotional support if they develop this female-dominated condition.

Breast cancer has increased quite dramatically in the West over the last 40 years or so, although the *rate* of increase has gradually levelled off over the last decade. This is probably at least partially due to reduced use of hormone replacement therapy (HRT) for menopausal symptoms. Many breast tumours are stimulated by these female hormones (oestrogen and progesterone). However, it's interesting to note that the combined rates of all types of cancer have also shown a similar pattern of rapid growth, followed by a more recent levelling off, so there may be some other influences which are affecting cancer in general.

This is potentially good news, but one in eight women in the UK will still develop breast cancer at some time during their lives.

However, more people who get breast cancer are surviving it. Nowadays, according to Cancer Research UK, 78% of women in the UK survive at least ten years from their diagnosis, and nearly two thirds survive beyond 20 years. In comparison, in the 1970s, only 40% would still be alive after ten years.

These improved survival rates may be somewhat overestimated, as breast screening can pick up small tumours, some of which may never otherwise have gone on to become troublesome. (Sometimes our body's own defences can deal with small tumours, although this is never a reason to ignore any lumps or other breast changes.) Nevertheless, detecting breast cancer earlier through screening has undoubtedly had a genuinely positive effect on survival, as early treatment is important.

There is also an overall trend for improved survival from all cancers since the 1970s, and this is probably due to earlier diagnosis allowing earlier treatment, as well as improvements in treatment for some forms of cancer.

Summary:

Cancer cells look and act abnormally, and ignore the body's signal to stop growing. Cancers grow by the cells doubling, so the more cancer cells there are, the faster the tumour appears to grow.

We all have cancer cells in our body from time to time, but usually our immune system destroys them.

Breast cancer can affect both sexes.

The main types are ductal (from the milk ducts) or lobular (from the breast lobules).

DCIS is a condition where breast cells look abnormal but have not yet become cancerous.

Cancer rates (both overall and for breast cancer specifically) have been increasing over recent decades, however the rate of increase has started to tail off in recent years.

Decreased use of HRT by women has probably contributed to this tailing off.

Earlier diagnosis is probably responsible for some of the improved survival rates seen for many cancers over recent years.

Further Information:

Cancer Research UK	http://goo.gl/6QEO6b
National Cancer Institute	http://goo.gl/tdhfVq
Breast Cancer Now	http://goo.gl/sdvytO

Dr Susan Love's Breast Book: S M Love with K Lindsey – Da Capo

Act with Love	http://goo.gl/2Pwjo1
The Guardian	http://goo.gl/QuGGkC

Chapter 3

What do you do if something is wrong with your breasts?

First, have a very low threshold for suspicion. Breast cancer doesn't always appear as a hard golf-ball in your breast, with a flag sticking out of it saying 'Make an appointment with your doctor — now'.

It may surprise you that I didn't even notice the 5 cm diameter lump in my right breast, nor did my GP. So if anything about your breast just doesn't seem "right", go to your doctor and ask to be assessed by a Breast Specialist.

My Story

I slid open the shower door and shivered as I stepped onto the bath mat. Grabbing the dark blue bath towel, I glanced in the mirror as I wrapped it around me.

The glance turned to a stare. There was a patch of red on my right breast. My towel dropped to the floor. I froze, all thoughts of the day forgotten. Deep inside, a whirlpool of fear began to spin.

No, it's OK — probably just the hot shower water.

But the red patch had a definite edge. It wasn't right.

I walked into my small bright bedroom, lay down on the bedspread and felt my breasts carefully all over. I couldn't feel any lumps. I felt deep into both armpits - no swollen lymph glands. Calm, professional, logical — sick with fear.

I took a deep breath and stared at the ceiling. A small black spider scuttled towards the corner. I must get the duster to that web.

But, what about this red patch?

I took a deep breath. OK. I'll keep an eye on it. If it doesn't disappear, I'll —

think what to do …

But after the next shower that red mark was still there — no bigger, no smaller — just there. And after every subsequent shower it was the same …

A couple of weeks later I went for a bra-fitting. A nice opportunity to treat myself to a pretty bra, which fitted perfectly. This time it was different though. As I stood in the small dark cubicle, I was aware that the pleasant middle-aged assistant was looking increasingly puzzled as she hunched in front of me, her hand delving deep into the bra I was trying.

'Your left breast fits perfectly Madam, but I'm having real trouble with the right one. There's something not quite right.'

This had never happened before. The small cubicle was stifling now, I felt hot, couldn't breathe — I just wanted to get out. After an age she was finished and, clutching my new bra, I escaped into the street.

The cold air hit me, people barged past me, I stumbled into a tall man. He glared and hurried on. I felt dizzy. A coffee would help. I pushed on the heavy door of the coffee shop next door. The noise was deafening. I clutched the counter as I waited in the long queue. Finally there was just one more woman in front of me. She started to order…

'A skinny latte with whipped cream, marshmallows and extra chocolate.'

'Anything else?'

'Are those toasties cheese or ham?'

'They're tuna.'

'Tuna? Oh I don't know if I fancy tuna. What's in those croissants?'

'Cheese and ham'

'Oh, and what about these?'

The room was spinning now as she dallied over which particular piece of junk food she needed to keep starvation at bay between lunch and dinner.

Eventually she settled on a low fat pasta salad and a large chocolate brownie.

I ordered a small Americano and carried it to the only free table — small, coffee-stained, with wobbly legs, squashed between two groups of boisterous women.

I placed the drink, half of which was by now in the saucer, on the tiny table and sat down on the hard chair. I took a sip, then a deep breath, all the time trying to collect my thoughts. I put my hand over my ear to muffle the screams of laughter from the table to my left.

'Oops, sorry.' One of the women had stood up suddenly, without checking what was in the path of her generous derrière. I just managed to save the last of my coffee as she knocked my table again, shoving it four inches nearer the door. I poured the coffee from my saucer back into the cup and tried again to think straight.

I'd had a red patch on my breast for a couple of weeks now — almost always there, always in the same place, always the same shape. It looked innocent enough, just slightly flushed skin. I'd felt my breast repeatedly and couldn't find any lumps, but now the bra-fitter had commented that my breast wasn't right. She spends all day feeling boobs. I should trust her judgment.

It was no good, I would have to see my GP. He'd probably say I was being neurotic — after all, doctors usually are when it comes to themselves, but best to get it checked.

Having made the decision I relaxed a little. I drank the dregs of my coffee, grabbing cup and saucer once more as the woman squeezed past my table on her return, then I got up and headed out.

I'll phone the surgery first thing tomorrow, I mumbled to myself as I opened the door into the street.

This is how my breast cancer announced itself, but it can appear in many ways.

The first thing people think of with breast cancer is a lump. Lumps can be small or large, soft, firm or hard, smooth or uneven. Some are filled with fluid (a cyst) and some are solid. Certain aspects of the lump make it more or less likely to be cancer. Either way, it's extremely important that any breast lump is checked out—and that means at least a visit to a breast specialist and usually some further tests such as a mammogram, ultrasound or biopsy.

Even breast surgeons, who spend all their working day examining women's chests — both on the outside and the inside — would rarely if ever say that a breast lump was definitely not cancer without doing further tests. Every now and then, a lump which has all the features of a benign (non-cancerous) lump is found to contain cancer cells, and it is so quick and easy nowadays to do some simple tests — so why wouldn't they? Early detection is always best.

Sometimes the lump isn't in the breast itself, but under the arm instead. There are two reasons for this: breast tissue actually extends quite a long way under the arm, or the lump may be an enlarged lymph node. Cancer cells can spread from the breast to the lymph nodes, which act as one of the body's defence systems against cancer and swell as they try to contain the cancer cells and prevent them spreading further. Sometimes they succeed, but sometimes the cancer cells break through this defence.

A breast can be quite firm, and is full of lobules, where the milk is produced, so it can be difficult to distinguish an abnormal lump from the normal tissue. There are various guides available on how to examine your breast properly, and these may help, but at the end of the day your doctor can give an experienced and unbiased opinion. Your GP should have a low threshold for sending you to see a breast specialist, and if you're concerned that they haven't, you must insist on a referral. Equally, just because they refer you doesn't necessarily mean you have cancer, they may be erring on the side of caution.

Sometimes you might discover something different about your breast. You may see changes in the nipple – it may have become inverted (turned in on itself). Some women's nipples are permanently inverted, and this is nothing to worry about. What is of concern is a change — if they become inverted when they weren't before. You may notice a rash around the nipple, or a discharge, or bleeding from the nipple, or a change in the nipple shape. Any of these findings require a prompt visit to your doctor.

Sometimes the breast is just a bit swollen for no good reason. Breasts can become swollen and/or painful, particularly before a period. This can be normal, but an unusual pain or swelling may need checking — especially if it only affects one breast.

As in my case, the skin of your breast may change. It may become thickened, or dimpled. Sometimes the skin take on the appearance of the skin of an orange and this is known by the French name *peau d'orange*. This is quite likely to be cancer and should *always* be checked.

However, your breasts can't read textbooks and sometimes they just do their own thing, so any skin change, or in fact any change in your breasts should be a reason to go to your doctor.

At the end of the day, you know your breasts better than anyone, and if you think something isn't quite right, it probably isn't. It may not be cancer, but it deserves investigation. One of the main reasons why you should check your breasts regularly is so that you can be more certain when something changes — but if life is busy and you haven't actually got down to that item on your 'to-do list' and find something wrong, don't worry, you're certainly not alone.

Summary:

Not all breast lumps are cancer — but some are, so always have them checked. Sometimes you may not feel a lump — check out any changes in your breast or under your arm.
Your GP should refer you to a breast specialist if there are any suspicions about your breasts.

Further Information:

Macmillan Cancer Support   http://goo.gl/9KtaL1
Cancer Research UK   http://goo.gl/RgFNeb
BreastCancer.Org   http://goo.gl/k6OyDW

13

Chapter 4

Breast screening

Breast screening (mammography, that is, breast x-rays) was introduced in the UK from the late eighties. Women aged 47 to 73 are currently offered screening. You may be offered breast screening at a younger age if you're at particular risk.

Screening appears to reduce the death rate from breast cancer, however there is some controversy about this. It may pick up tumours before women are aware of them, which means they're more likely to respond to treatment. However, some of these may never have developed into full-blown cancer, so over-diagnosis is a potential issue. Screening also involves radiation, which isn't totally without risk.

Some large studies have been undertaken to establish the true benefit of screening – including a Swedish study of 133,065 women. This concluded that, overall, survival improvements were still worthwhile.

As with many tests, the accuracy isn't 100%. Sometimes there'll be false positive results (where a cancer is wrongly diagnosed) or false negatives (where a cancer is missed by screening) — often in younger women, who have denser breast tissue.

Although a false positive is of course worrying, further investigations should establish that there isn't any cancer. Missed cancers are more of a problem, because a woman may be wrongly reassured, meaning that she fails to seek medical help when she experiences symptoms. Breast cancer is missed on around 20% of screening mammograms, so even if you've recently had a clear mammogram, please do see your doctor if anything is wrong.

If something abnormal is detected, or if there are technical problems, you may be recalled for further assessment. This doesn't automatically mean that you have cancer. In fact only around one in six women who are called back turn out to have cancer.

If you're having treatment for breast cancer, your GP should inform the Screening Unit to prevent them inviting you for a screening mammography at that time.

Five years after your breast cancer treatment has finished, you will revert back into the breast screening program for your regular mammograms. If you don't receive an invitation at this point, do contact your GP or cancer specialist and make sure you get one.

Summary:

Screening can diagnose breast cancer early, thereby improving chances of cure and allowing an easier treatment regime.

Screening may also pick up tumours which may never have become a problem.

Screening involves X-raying the breasts every three years, thus exposing the women to extra irradiation.

The benefits of screening probably outweigh the downsides.

Screening isn't 100% accurate, so if you think something isn't right, see your doctor — even if you've recently had a normal mammogram.

During cancer treatment, and for a period of time afterwards (usually 5 years), you'll be monitored by your breast unit. Afterwards you should be monitored via the breast screening programme once more.

Further Information:

NHS Breast Screening Programme	http://goo.gl/JjPTU1
Cancer Research UK	http://goo.gl/Of7M6w
NHS Choices	http://bit.ly/1RoMz4z
National Cancer Institute	http://goo.gl/SP0VD4

"Swedish two-county trial: impact of mammographic screening on breast cancer mortality during 3 decades". Tabár L et al, *Radiology.* 2011 Sep; 260(3): pages 658–63.
http://goo.gl/NlbDXY

"Absolute numbers of lives saved and overdiagnosis in breast cancer screening, from a randomized trial and from the Breast Screening Programme in England". Duffy S.W. et al, *J Med Screen.* 2010; 17(1): pages 25–30
http://goo.gl/HksSQd

Chapter 5

The Breast Unit

If there's any possibility that you have breast cancer, your GP should refer you to a Breast Unit. These are specialist units where professionals who specialize in breast diseases, including cancer, work closely together. It's an efficient set-up, designed to provide the best care.

In England at the time of writing, whether or not cancer is suspected, you should be seen within two weeks of your GP's referral — as recommended by Department of Health guidelines. Time-frames are similar in the rest of the UK.

Breast Units vary operationally, but you should be seen and examined by a breast specialist. You may only need the doctor's examination. He may be able to reassure you that all's fine and send you home. However, breast units are able to offer other tests, which you may or may not need, for example mammography and ultrasound examinations.

This is what happened to me at my first visit ...

My Story

The middle-aged receptionist was half hidden behind a pile of notes. Phone cradled to her ear, she checked my name on a torn sheet of A4 sellotaped to the desk.

Putting a hand over the phone she said, 'Down the corridor. You'll be called for a mammogram.'

Mammogram? I thought I was coming to see the breast specialist? I opened my mouth with the question, but she was deep in conversation again. I wandered in the direction she'd indicated. The long narrow corridor opened into a huge, bright waiting room. Piles of magazines lay on numerous small tables, surrounded by plastic chairs and small sofas.

I noticed the magazines looked quite new – ah well, I might as well enjoy the wait with some guilt-free relaxation and a quiet read. I found a seat and took off my coat and jumper. I started talking to myself (a bad habit of mine). I told myself that this was good for me, experiencing what cancer patients go through. Doctors didn't often get this chance. Obviously — thankfully — it'd only be a superficial insight, because I didn't actually have cancer.

I picked up a magazine, and soon I was absorbed in an article about a Pacific island fruit which caused remarkable weight loss and apparently tasted delicious too. I jotted down the fruit's name for later.

'Kathleen Thompson?' A female voice sliced through my concentration. Flinging down the half-read article, I grabbed bag, coat and jumper and hurried after the disappearing white uniform into a small changing room. Minutes later I was stripped to the waist and wearing a starched blue gown that opened down the front, standing in a room with a large X-ray machine.

'OK, could you undo your gown please? I need to position your breast between these two perspex plates. It's a bit awkward, and it'll feel uncomfortable, but it'll soon be over.' The young radiographer smiled reassurance as she guided me boob-first towards the cold metal machine.

Then followed a bizarre game of Twister as she manipulated my body into the ungainly position necessary for the mammogram. Eventually, my right breast was squashed to her satisfaction, between the two plates, and resembled a partially deflated beach ball. She scurried behind the lead-lined wall to the controls, shouting over her shoulder that I should keep very still. This last instruction seemed redundant, as any movement could only have been achieved by leaving a valued part of my anatomy behind in the perspex vice.

A few seconds later, the X-ray plates moved apart and my breast was reunited with the rest of me. She repeated the pantomime to secure my left one. As the plates squeezed once again I worried about my breast ligaments. Would they be stretched and damaged? The fight against age was a constant battle, and my body didn't need an extra shove along the downhill spiral.

The x-ray over, I checked that my breasts were still attached to my body, dressed and returned to the waiting room, found a seat and tried to read, but this time I couldn't concentrate.

A voice close-by startled me, 'If they see anything suspicious on your mammogram, they'll do an ultrasound examination.' I looked up and saw a nurse was talking to a young blond woman sitting next to me.

Just then, another nurse appeared from the X-ray department. She walked towards me, her black lace-ups squeaking.

'Kathleen Thompson?'

'Yes.'

She pirouetted and headed off in the opposite direction. I jumped up, grabbed my belongings like a deranged bag lady, and jogged after her.

She led me into a small dark room. I could just make out a large metal instrument by a couch at the far side. I recognized it as an ultrasound machine.

I replayed the conversation I'd just overheard, 'If they see anything suspicious on your mammogram, they'll do an ultrasound examination'.

So they must have seen something, and they're going to do an ultrasound, and probably they'll take a biopsy too. My doctor head was matter-of-fact, logical and calm, but the woman in me was screaming. No — this isn't meant to happen. There must be some mistake.

Everything had taken on a strange quality — like a dream. That's what it was—just a bad nightmare. Surely I'd wake up in a minute, covered in sweat, snuggled under my duvet?

From Both Ends Of The Stethoscope

Summary:

GPs should send women with breast changes to a Breast Unit.
Your appointment should be within 2 weeks.
You'll see a specialist doctor (breast surgeon), and may or may not have tests
including mammography, ultrasound examination and biopsy.
These may all happen on the same day.

Further Information:

Breast Cancer Care   http://goo.gl/ZFnTMp
Cancer Research UK   http://goo.gl/Vv4v6V

20

Chapter 6

Initial tests (mammogram, ultrasound, biopsy)

Breast Units have specialist radiologists, who are experts in breast cancer imaging. I attended a Breast Unit where they were able to perform a mammogram on my first visit and read it within a few minutes. When they saw a suspicious area, they were able to perform an ultrasound immediately and take a biopsy sample. This meant that I could leave the clinic with a very good idea of what was wrong, and just had to wait for the pathology report of the biopsy for confirmation.

My Story

The nurse asked me to lie on the couch by the ultrasound machine.
'The doctor will be here soon.'
A tall man with white hair walked through the door and smiled. He sat down next to the machine.
Looking straight into my eyes, he spoke, 'The problem is, we've seen a lump on your X-ray. So I need to look at it with this ultrasound.'
Very gently, he pulled down my blue gown and exposed my breasts. I flinched as he squirted a blob of cold gel onto my skin. He pressed the ultrasound probe onto the blob and moved it slowly over my right breast for a few minutes. He pointed to the fuzzy image on the small screen.
'This is the lump. It's about 2cm wide.' His voice was quiet but firm. 'Do you see the irregular shape, and these little bright flecks? These are worrying.'
He looked at me as he said this. His blue eyes sent sympathy and strength.
The screen looked like an ancient TV with a lousy reception. I couldn't make

21

out any lump, but I understood 'irregular shape' and 'worrying' well enough.

'I notice you're a doctor — where do you practice?' he continued.

'I was a paediatrician, but now I work in drug research.'

'Oh? Interesting.' His smile morphed into a more serious expression, 'I need to take a biopsy of this lump. We have these neat little things now.' He held a small black box between his finger and thumb.

'I'm going to press this box over the lump, then push this button, and a needle will shoot out and take the sample. It'll make a loud click, but it won't hurt, because I'm going to numb you first.'

I lay on the couch in the semi-darkness, watching him fill a small syringe with local anaesthetic. The coldness of the wall, pressing against my left arm, forced me to concentrate. Everything was unreal — surreal. What was I doing here? I only came for a check. My left hand gripped the coarse material of the hospital gown, as if it was a survival rope. My right hand was visible to him and the nurse, so I forced it to relax.

Lifting the small syringe towards me, he injected the anaesthetic into my breast. It stung, but I hid the pain with a smile. 'No, it doesn't hurt. It's fine. A lovely day outside. I don't expect you'll have much chance to enjoy it, stuck in here.'

Somehow I controlled my voice, but tears were streaming down my face. I hoped the darkened room would hide them.

Then, a loud click shattered the quiet. He'd taken the biopsy, and he was right, it hadn't hurt.

'Well done. All finished. Nurse will pop a dressing on for you. Then she'll take you to see the breast surgeon. Good luck with your research work.' And he was gone.

A mammogram can sometimes detect a lump that you haven't felt. The edge of the lump and its shape can offer a clue as to whether or not it's cancer. If it's smooth-edged and round, it may be an innocent cyst, but if it's an odd shape with uneven or jagged edges, it's more likely to be cancer. Having said this, a doctor would normally do further tests to make absolutely sure — for example he may take a biopsy or, for a fluid-filled cyst, a sample of the fluid to test it for cancer cells.

Sometimes breast lumps contain calcified areas, which appear white on the X-ray. Larger calcified areas can appear as people get older, and these are less worrying, but if the lump has lots of tiny specks of calcium, this often indicates that there are actively dividing cells in the area — which means cancer.

An ultrasound machine uses high frequency sound waves to create a picture of the body's internal organs. It works on the same principle as submarines (and bats), using sonar. It's useful for looking at parts of the body that aren't covered in bone, and provides more — and different — information than the mammogram.

I hadn't felt a breast lump myself, but one had been seen on my mammogram and that's why I was given an ultrasound examination after the mammogram.

Summary:

When you go for your first appointment at a Breast Unit, you will see a doctor.
You may have various tests including mammogram and/or ultrasound.
If a lump is found in your breast a doctor will probably take a biopsy or some fluid
from it to check whether there is any cancer present.

Further Information:

Breast Cancer Care   http://goo.gl/ZFnTMp
Office on Women's Health   http://goo.gl/tcyHht

Chapter 7

The health professionals in a breast unit

Breast Units house staff of various disciplines, specialising in breast disease in general and breast cancer in particular. These include surgeons, nurses, radiologists and radiographers. There are also other specialists in the background, such as pathologists who are experienced in examining breast biopsies.

Breast Surgeon

At some point during your assessment you should see a doctor who specializes in treating breast diseases. This person will usually be a surgeon. They spend their days dealing with breast problems — not just cancer, but benign (non-cancerous) lumps, and other abnormalities. They're very skilled at assessing breast lumps and at operating on breasts, and many of them have plastic surgery training too. The breast is closely associated with body image for many women, and the loss of a breast, or even the removal of a large lump, can have a devastating psychological effect.

Women in the UK are lucky. We have access to many excellent breast surgeons and plastic surgeons who have developed skillful operations that minimize the effects on a woman's appearance. In fact breasts can sometimes look better after cancer surgery than they did before — although this hardly compensates for having breast cancer.

When you first meet the surgeon, they will examine you, and may reassure you that everything is normal (the preferred option). However, they may tell you that you need some more tests, especially if they feel a lump. Alternatively they may indicate to you that it is highly likely you have cancer. All this

25

depends on what they find when they examine you. Doctors and nurses try to be as honest as possible and give you as much information as they can. Sometimes, though, they simply cannot answer all of your questions until they have more information.

Breast Care Nurse
The breast care nurses, or nurse practitioners as some prefer to be called, specialise in helping patients with breast cancer, or suspected breast cancer, and provide help and support throughout the cancer treatment. As in most professions, individual nurses vary. Most are absolute angels, treating each person as if they are the most important patient in the clinic, listening and responding with patience and practicality to all the many crazy worries that flood into a person's mind as soon as the dams of reason are smashed by the words "You have cancer". Many work tirelessly, knowing that what might be just another day in the office for them is a personal devastation for every patient they encounter, as well as for their close relatives/friends.

Of course not all breast care nurses achieve these superhuman standards. Some occasionally give inappropriate advice or are unhelpful. I have encountered both types. If you are concerned, don't be frightened to insist on seeing the doctor directly.

Eileen, the Breast Care Nurse who I encountered on that first hospital visit was definitely one of God's Angels.

Radiologists and Radiographers
A radiologist is a doctor who specializes in images (X-ray, MRI or Ultrasound) and a radiographer is trained in the technical side of actually producing the images. Specialist radiographers also work in the radiotherapy department, because the skills required to provide radiotherapy are similar to those needed for taking X-rays.

My Story

After the biopsy, I followed the nurse back outside. There were some chairs in the corridor. A young couple occupied two of them. They both had dark hair, and he wore a football top covered in Italian writing.

'Sit down here for a minute. Someone will come and take you to the doctor.' The nurse indicated a chair then walked away.

Reluctantly, I sat down opposite the couple. My tears were unstoppable now. I kept my head bent low, pretending to be searching for something in my handbag.

The radiologist hadn't told me in so many words that I had cancer, but I was no fool. He'd told me the appearance of the lump was irregular and that it was worrying. I knew this wasn't likely to be a benign cyst. From his manner I knew he was sure it was cancer.

'Lucia Williams?' The woman opposite stood up. The man stayed sitting as his wife followed the nurse through another door.

I continued to study the pattern on the lining of my handbag as if the meaning of life was hidden within its shapes.

'I'm going for a cup of tea, would you like one?' his voice was friendly.

'No, thanks I'm fine.' I mumbled towards the zip at the top of my bag.

Whilst he was gone I quickly found a paper tissue and wiped my wet face, blew my nose and took a few deep breaths. I dug out my i-phone and checked my face in the camera app. Was it obvious I'd been crying?

He returned carrying a small plastic cup and sat down again.

I had to say something — mustn't appear rude. My face felt dry now, maybe I could risk looking up?

'I noticed your football top. Are you Italian?'

He smiled. 'Actually this is a famous Italian rugby team. My wife is Italian and we used to live out there. Then she got multiple sclerosis, so we decided to come back to England for her medical care. Our eldest was just coming up to five, so it seemed sensible to move back before he started school. Then she found this breast lump.'

'Oh, you must be so worried. How is your wife feeling?'

He paused.

'She'll probably be crying when she comes out. Just like you, and just like the woman who was sitting there before you'.

His gentle remark touched me deeply. It made me realize that I wasn't the first, and wouldn't be the last person to weep in this department. I also learned that my little handbag trick hadn't fooled anyone.

We chatted like old comrades. I explained that my ex-husband, who was still a good friend, was half-Italian and we laughed as we swapped amusing stories about life in Italy. For a moment I forgot the enormity of my situation.

A door creaked open and his wife came out slowly and sat next to him. She seemed upset,

'How was it?' *he asked, as he put his arm round her shoulders.*

'That woman really 'urt me, doing that … what is it? Biopsy?

'She said I 'ave to see the doctor now, but I thought she was the doctor?'

'She is a doctor, she'll have been one of the radiologists. Now you need to see the surgeon. It's a different doctor.' *She stared at my interruption blankly, as I tried to explain to her. It made me realize that, scary though this was, at least hospitals were familiar territory to me.*

Then I heard an Irish accent. 'Kathleen Thompson?'

It startled me. I hadn't noticed the petite lady approach.

She was smiling at me. Late fifties, tall, slim, grey hair and blue eyes, dressed in 'civvies' — a knee-length brown skirt and pale-blue jumper.

'I'm Eileen, one of the breast care nurses. Let's go in and see the surgeon and then we can have a chat.'

'Hello, hello. Sit down.' *The surgeon waved a plump hand to the seat in front of his desk.*

'So we've found a breast lump? Let's take a look.'

For the third time in two hours, I stripped to the waist and lay on yet another couch. He examined my breasts clumsily. I knew how a breast should be examined and was bewildered at the half-hearted grope by this apparent expert.

When he'd finished I dressed and followed him to the desk.

'Have you any questions?' *he asked as he sat down and started writing notes.*

'What happens next?'

'Well I can't tell you until we have the biopsy results. I've already told you everything I can.'

'Then, no … no more questions.' *As I stared at him, not sure what else to say, I felt a gentle hand on my arm. It was Nurse Eileen.*

'Come on dear.' *She led me out of the consulting room. She chatted to me constantly whilst guiding me down a corridor. Then she stopped and opened a door into a bright, cheerful room, carpeted in pale pink. A small, cream, cottage-style chintz sofa and two matching chairs made the room look cosy. A box of tissues was discretely placed on the glass-topped, light wood table. The room seemed out of place — an attempt at a comfortable oasis within the sterile hospital environment.*

'Come and sit down, dear. It's quieter in here.'

I noticed she was studying my reaction. I guessed that this room had been her idea. To be honest, I didn't care whether the room looked cheerful or utilitarian, it didn't alter anything. I suppose my lack of response must have disappointed her.

'Now then, how do you take your tea?'

'Just black, no sugar.'

'OK, back in a mo.'

I sat on the chintz sofa and waited for her.

I was numb now, past crying. I helped myself to a clean tissue, putting my saturated one in the wicker wastepaper bin. I looked around the room, but didn't really see anything.

Eileen came back with a plastic cup of tea and a small plate of biscuits.

Bizarre disjointed thoughts popped into my mind: Did anyone ever eat those biscuits? OMG, I've got breast cancer, but never mind that, those look like choccy digestives. My favourites. I wonder if I can take two?

I tried to suppress my crazy thoughts and focus on what Eileen was saying.

Her Irish lilt reminded me of the nuns when I was in school. It felt warm, reassuring. I was no longer a professional. I wanted to be a child again surrounded by adults who would keep me safe. More than anything I didn't want to have to think for myself or make important decisions, particularly the ones which I would need to make soon, and which would shape my whole future.

'The doctor you just saw was the registrar. Don't worry, when you come back next time Miss Gomez will be here. She's the consultant and I'll make sure you see her.'

She spoke as if, of all the patients passing through the clinic, I was somehow special, and she would champion my case.

I couldn't speak, but she filled the silence with quiet conversation. She paused, then commented, almost to herself,

'It's so hard when you're sitting there looking the picture of health and feeling so fit and well ...' At the time I didn't really understand the full implication of what she stopped herself from saying.

'Here take these booklets dear. Breast Cancer Care produce them. I know you're a doctor, but you may still find them useful. They go through the different sorts of breast cancer and the treatments. Take them with you and have a quiet read. It's a lot to take in at the moment.'

'What will happen next?'

She paused, as if thinking how to reply. 'Well it depends on what the biopsy shows. I think you will definitely need to have the lump removed. You may need radiotherapy too, if it is cancer, and you might need chemotherapy. We'll know for sure when we have your results.'

She probably said a lot more things too, but I didn't hear them.

'OK, let's get you home. I'll take you to the car park through a back corridor, it'll be quieter.' She didn't say that it wouldn't do me or the other waiting patients a lot of good for them to witness my tears, which had started up once again, but I suspect it had crossed her mind.

I followed her through a maze of deserted corridors, then she opened a fire exit door, and we were in the car park.

'Take my business card, Kathleen. If you think of anything else you need to ask just call me or email me. If I'm not there when you phone, I'll get back to you quickly.' We hugged like old friends.

'Are you OK to drive?'

'Oh yes, I'm fine! Thanks Eileen. You've been so kind. I'm really grateful.' And I was.

Summary:

Breast Units house staff of various disciplines, who specialize in breast disease in general and breast cancer in particular.

They will try to tell you what they can, but may not know everything until they have done more tests.

Further Information:

Breast Cancer Care   http://goo.gl/ZFnTMp

Chapter 8

What does it feel like when you find out you have cancer?

The word Cancer is evocative in the extreme. When I was a newly-qualified doctor, the medical profession used a series of euphemisms for it. This way, we could talk about a patient's illness in front of them, without them understanding the horror of what we were saying. First we called it carcinoma, but when this word became more generally recognized for what it was, we switched to neoplasia — always one step ahead of public knowledge. Just thirty years on, this behaviour is totally unacceptable, and quite rightly. Doctors and other medical staff are expected to be as frank and honest as possible with their patients. At the time, though, we truly believed we were being kind.

We weren't alone. People didn't talk about their cancer either. It was hushed up as something too shocking to share. Many people didn't even know they had cancer; their relatives would be told, but they would be kept in the dark.

This made the Cancer Demon even bigger and more scary than it actually was, because the only time people knew someone had cancer was when they were about to die or had already died. This compounded the myth that cancer was always a death sentence.

It's important to understand that although people do die of this disease, by no means everyone does. Some cancers can be cured, and even where they're not cured, one can often continue to lead a full and active life for many years.

Many people still don't know this though, or if they know it at an intellectual level, it still hasn't sunk in at an emotional one. Deep in our psyche, cancer is

32

synonymous with Death, Suffering, Pain, Horror and Hopelessness. People's experiences of learning they have cancer will differ, influenced partly by circumstances, past experiences and individual personalities. However, human reaction to extremely difficult situations has been researched, and it seems that there are some common threads.

Elisabeth Kübler-Ross, an American psychiatrist, interviewed many patients with terminal illness. Her book On Death and Dying, published in 1969, talks about different stages that people go through when faced with death. These have become known as the Five Stages of Grief, because we now realise that people go through these stages in many catastrophic life situations such as bereavement, or finding out that they have a life-threatening disease.

Knowledge of these stages can help us understand people's occasionally bizarre reactions to extremely bad news, and can also give us insight into our own behaviour.

Kübler-Ross named the five stages:

Stage 1: Denial and Isolation
Stage 2: Anger
Stage 3: Bargaining
Stage 4: Depression
Stage 5: Acceptance

These stages are normal, and the hope is that people will work their way through them all until they finally reach an acceptance of their situation. However, people in terrible situations haven't always attended a How-to-Behave-in-Dire-Situations course and (as Kübler-Ross herself realised), they don't always go through the stages in neat order, or at all. Sometimes they skip stages, or go back and forth between them, and some people become permanently stuck and never achieve acceptance.

The Denial stage is very common — a feeling of disbelief: 'There must be some mistake'. People may demand second, third and fourth opinions. At a subconscious level most of us consider ourselves immortal — dying is something that happens to other people. Sometimes the news is accepted on one level, whilst denial is demonstrated in other ways, such as terminally ill patients making future plans which are blatantly unrealistic.

Anger can follow closely on from denial, or co-exist with it. People may become angry with their doctors, accusing them of delay in diagnosis or poor care; angry with God or with someone who they feel may have contributed to their illness; angry with other people who are fit and well. 'Why me? Look at him, he's smoked all his life, stuffed himself with pies and beer and he's over eighty and still here. Bloody not fair.' Someone with cancer may become unreasonably angry with people close to them — who naturally will be confused and upset by this reaction. It's important to understand that this anger isn't 'personal', it's just the result of someone struggling to deal with an impossible situation, and sometimes the people closest are the easiest target.

The Bargaining stage is just what it says: 'God, just let me live until my daughter's wedding', 'Just give me one more year God', 'If I give up smoking, let me get better' and so on.

Eventually, as realization sinks in, Depression replaces the numbness of denial and the anger and hopeful bargaining. There are many obvious reasons why someone faced with devastation will be depressed, and this stage is necessary as the person faces the true realization of their situation.

Ideally, if someone has had the time and support to work through the stages successfully, they will start to accept their fate, without denial or anger. It's possible to lose even the fear of death — trust me, I did. For those who get stuck in a stage though, experienced counselling may be helpful.

It is important to remember too, that it isn't just the person with cancer who's going through the grief process. Their friends and loved ones will be experiencing the grief of having someone close to them suffering from cancer too, and they may react strangely due to their own denial or anger. It is important to understand this.

So that's the theory, and now I'd like to share some of my personal experiences with you.

My Story

I was not fine though.

I sat in my car. What should I do? Everything was so very different from the last time I'd sat there, just a couple of hours earlier. How was I going to drive home? I was shaking, trying to think straight. Someone tapped on my window to ask if I was vacating the parking space. No. Not yet. Leave me alone. Can't you see I'm falling apart?

But of course they couldn't. My life had changed irreversibly, yet all around me other people's lives were going on as if nothing extraordinary had happened.

34

I had to fix on something. I desperately needed a familiar face, someone to talk to. My kids were both at work. I couldn't upset them. I hadn't told anyone I was here today. I hadn't really expected they'd find anything wrong.

I remembered I had some bubble-wrap in the boot of my car. It was there because I had planned to drop it into Phil, my ex-boyfriend. That's what I'd do. I'd take Phil the bubble-wrap.

I reversed out of the space gingerly, narrowly missing the wing of the mini next to me as I swung out.

BEEEEEP.

Oh my God, where did that car come from? I braked, changed into first and edged forward like a novice, ignoring the revving of the car behind me, which seemed to be riveted to my rear bumper. The scowl of its driver was clearly visible in my rearview mirror.

Somehow I negotiated my way through the busy town centre and reached Phil's house. As I pulled up I saw him moving around in his tiny kitchen. Thank God, he was home. I got out of my car, walked up the short path and knocked on the front door. There was no reply. I looked through the window. The kitchen appeared empty now. I knocked again – louder.

After a few more minutes I saw his shape through the frosted glass. He opened the door very slowly. 'Oh, hello – it's you.'

'Hi. I've brought the bubble-wrap.'

'Oh, yeah, thanks.'

He took it from me and paused, hand on the front door. Our 'let's be friends' strategy hadn't been going too smoothly of late. It was more like armed neutrality with a bubbling undercurrent of emotion — sometimes détente, sometimes Cold War.

Perhaps I shouldn't have come. I stood motionless on the doorstep. I couldn't walk away. I couldn't think. I couldn't drive. I was numb, shocked, confused.

'Did you want a cup of tea?' he asked eventually.

'Yes. That would be nice.'

I stepped over his muddy running shoes and followed him into the familiar kitchen with its two bar stools. It was the only place in his house where we could sit. There was just a solitary reclining chair occupying his small lounge. I remembered how I used to grumble about that.

'Why did you want the bubble-wrap?'

'Oh, I'm sending a commemorative mug to Nick. It's the centenary of his sports

club, *before he moved to Oz. I thought he might like it.'*

'I'm sure he will. You must miss him.'

'I do, but he phones me every week and we're in touch by email all the time.'

'Well remember me to him next time, won't you? And how's Tim? Is he OK?'

'Yes, he's fine.'

He answered my questions, but his lean face and pale blue eyes showed his perplexity as tears began to stream uncontrollably down my face. He passed me a steaming mug of tea, then, after taking a sip of his own, he moved his stool slightly further away and sat down. He folded his arms around his body and stared at me with defensive resignation.

I gazed at my mug. It was a souvenir of our holiday together at the Grand Canyon. I remembered how we'd walked up from the bottom in the heat.

His bar stool creaked as he shifted weight, and my memories scuttled away.

Should I explain why I was crying? Reassure him that it wasn't to do with him on this occasion? No, best not. There was no need to tell him I'd got cancer, it was nothing to do with him, not any more.

Even as I thought it, my mouth rebelled. 'I've just come from the hospital. I've got breast cancer.'

Before I'd finished blurting it out, he had leapt off his seat and put his arms round me. 'Don't worry,' he said, 'we'll get you through this'.

If you're reading this book before your first Breast Unit appointment, I would advise you not to do what I did. Tell someone you are going for the appointment, and ideally take someone with you. If everything is fine, that's great. But if it isn't fine, your whole life will have changed beyond recognition in minutes. Your head will be spinning, your emotions will be all over the place and you'll be as capable of driving as if you'd just been on every roller-coaster ride at Alton Towers, backwards. So, for your own safety, and that of innocent passers-by, it's good to have someone with you who can at least take the wheel. Actually, Liesel, a good friend of mine, had offered to come, but I was so convinced that everything would be fine, I'd refused. Big mistake.

My Story

When I returned home I made a cup of tea and sat down. I just felt so frightened. I kept repeating that overused question, 'Why me?'

I had been unexpectedly forced to face my own mortality, and the fact that it may be rushing towards me sooner than I'd thought. I'd been working hard on my diet and exercising. I was probably fitter, slimmer and younger-looking than I'd been for twenty years. I had more energy, and people were starting to remark how good I looked. I felt great.

So why had I received this shot across the bows of my happy little speedboat? Eileen thought that they might just remove the lump, but she'd also mentioned mastectomy. Now I had to face the possibility of disfiguring surgery and radiotherapy to my breasts.

Working as a paediatrican, and more recently as a pharmaceutical physician, it was many years since I'd treated adult patients, and I was unaware of the fantastic advances in restorative breast surgery. The mention of mastectomy sent my thoughts to the poor patients I'd seen many years ago, with one breast missing — just a flat chest where their womanhood used to be.

There had always been an un-traversable gulf in my mind between these women and me. Now I was facing the possibility that I may end up with this dreadful disfigurement too. I was no more immune to the ugliness of cancer than they had been.

Eileen had told me that I would need to take anti-oestrogen tablets, edging me rapidly into menopause. If my lymph nodes were affected I would also need chemotherapy. Despite the popular image of 'cancer victims' being waif-like, thin and emaciated, I knew that breast cancer treatment often caused weight gain. After all my hard work slimming, was I doomed to balloon into a menopausal whale?

Even as these thoughts bubbled up in my mind, I felt ashamed of my shallowness and tried to suppress them. The medical world was poised to save me from a slow and painful premature death from cancer, and all I could do was whine about the effects on my appearance.

But the thoughts refused to be suppressed. It was a very bad night.

My focus on the superficial was a feature of my denial, ignoring the real problem that I may die. I almost certainly had cancer. The doctors and nurses knew it, and I knew it too. The appearance of the lump on my mammogram was typical, even without the biopsy results. But I had no idea how bad it was. What were my prospects? Even though I was a doctor, and should have known better, I still associated cancer with death. You may feel better for a while, may even fool yourself that you're cured — but once the monster gets you it never lets go completely.

I know now that this is simply not true, but I spent a long night in the land of anguish and hopelessness. I thought of my kids in a world without me. The grandchildren I would never hold. I wondered how long I actually had.

Most of the staff at the hospital had been great. In particular, the radiologist who'd gently broken the news and taken the biopsy, and Eileen, who'd mothered me and reassured me as much as she was able. The surgeon hadn't been that great, but he was relatively junior, filling in for the consultant. I can see they were all in a quandary. On one hand they could hardly discuss my outlook before the cancer was confirmed, and without knowing the exact nature of it, it would have been impossible to give a reliable assessment of my survival chances. But if someone had just told me that even if I had cancer it didn't necessarily mean I would die; if someone had told me that nearly two thirds of women with breast cancer survive beyond 20 years; if someone had just told me these things, I may have slept a lot better that first night, and the subsequent ones. Sure, they couldn't talk about my specific case, but yes, there was hope.

If you are having problems dealing with the overwhelming feelings and fear after being told you have cancer, there's a useful book written by Val Sampson and Debbie Fenlon (see below). Val has had breast cancer herself, and Debbie is a breast care nurse. They give concise, practical advice on how to deal with your emotions.

Summary:

Despite improving rates of cancer survival, most people still assume cancer means death.
Two-thirds of women with breast cancer survive for longer than 20 years.
When faced with a devastating situation of any kind, people generally go through '5 Stages of Grief': Denial/isolation; Anger; Bargaining; Depression; Acceptance.
Take someone with you who could drive you home when you first attend the Breast Unit.

Further Information:

Book: On Death and Dying by E. Kübler-Ross published Scribner 1969
http://goo.gl/zRNtOV

Book: The Breast Cancer Book by V. Sampson and D Fenlon. Vermilion 2000

Chapter 9

How do you tell people that you have cancer?

The short answer is, not like I did …

My Story

I got back from Phil's house and started with a cup of tea. Then I raided my small drinks cupboard. There wasn't much in there, but I found a litre bottle of sherry, which my aunt had given me when I'd visited her.

I wanted to phone my kids and give them the news, but I wasn't sure how. I'd never had to do anything like this before, and besides, telling anyone just seemed to reaffirm that it was real.

I grabbed a glass from the kitchen (a little too large for sherry, but what the hell?) and poured a generous measure.

Several glasses later (or, to be accurate, one complete bottle of sherry later), after not knowing how to tell anyone my news, I wanted to talk.

I wanted my kids to know but I phoned my ex-husband first.

'Is there anything you need? Can I help? Do you want taking to hospital? Just call if you do, you know I'll help.'

'Thanks, I'm OK. Phil is taking me to the hospital, but I appreciate the offer. I need to tell the kids.'

'Do you want me to tell them?'

'No. I want to, but I thought I should warn you first in case they speak to you.'

'Yes of course. Don't forget, let me know if we can help.'

Then I phoned my two children. I didn't know what to say. As a mother, I wanted to protect them from the pain and worry of my serious and frightening illness. As time went on I shared more of my problems and fears with them, but in those early stages I found it very hard to discard the image I'd created for myself of superhuman parent, and show my vulnerability. I disregarded the fact that they were actually mature and responsible adults themselves.

'Hi Mickie, How are you? How's Ed?'

'Fine. What's wrong Mum?' My daughter hates talking on the phone, so she knew that either I'd had a computer catastrophe and urgently required her IT skills, or it was something else important.

'Oh nothing ... well ... I went to the hospital today ...'

'And?' She wasn't going to let me get away with small talk.

'Well, probably nothing to worry about, but they found a breast lump. I have to wait for the pathology results before I know if it's anything important. I'm going back to the hospital the week after next.'

'Oh, you OK?'

'Yes I'm fine. Anyway I just thought I'd let you know.'

'You feeling alright?'

'Yes, I'm fine.'

'Let me know if you need anything.'

'Yes, will do.

'OK Mum. Take care. Let me know what happens.'

So I'd told my daughter, it wasn't that hard. She didn't say much, but I could hear the concern in her voice. Now it was time to phone my son.

'Hi Mum, how are you?'

'I'm good, Joe, how are you?'

'Fine. How was your trip?'

'Not too bad — tiring. Joe, I had to go to the hospital today. They found a small breast lump.'

'Oh, Mum, why didn't you say? Are you OK? What does it mean?' I could hear the anxiety in his voice. I immediately panicked and back-pedalled furiously.

'Well, probably nothing to worry about, Joe. A lot of breast lumps are harmless. They took a sample and they're testing it, and I have to go back for the results the week after next. If it's anything abnormal they'll just remove it.'

'Oh, OK. Nothing to worry about? You sure?'

'No, no. Nothing to worry about.'

'Oh, that's good.' His voice revealed his relief. *'When do you go back to the hospital? I can take time off work to take you.'*

'That's kind Joe, but don't worry, Phil said he'd take me. I don't want you missing work.'

'Well, it's up to you Mum, but I'll take you if you need.'

'Thanks Joe, I know. Anyway how are you? What are you up to?'

'I'm fine. Charlotte's just come in so we're going out for dinner.'

'OK, Joe. Have a nice time. See you soon.'

'See you Mum.'

I'd watered down the information so much that he was left with the impression that I had a minor medical condition, something on a par with an ingrown toenail. Later, my ex-husband had to do what I had failed to do and explain the full implications to him. Joe wasn't a child, but my own inadequacies had made it difficult for me to speak the plain truth.

When and who you tell about your cancer is clearly a personal decision based on individual circumstances.

I found it difficult. Telling people made it more 'real', when all the time I was trying to retreat into my denial. I felt embarrassed to let people know that my breasts were defective. What if I needed a mastectomy? I didn't want people to know that I was minus a breast. Would men look at me in a different way? Would they visualise me with a defective chest? It was humiliating — too much to deal with.

Having gone through it, I can now say that it really does become easier when other people know, and from my experience, those close to you would prefer not to be 'protected'. But make sure you take it easy on yourself too. If you need time, take it. You're trying to readjust to a complete shift in everything you thought was normal about your life and your being. Allow yourself to be human.

It's best to be open and complete in the information you give people. Clearly there are special circumstances where you may need help — telling small children, for example. In this case it's worth getting professional help via your GP or the hospital, and a number of cancer websites also provide advice.

Most Breast Units can also give you information on support groups, which you may or may not find helpful.

You'll probably find that some days you feel like talking and some days you don't. You'll be happy to chat to some people about your cancer, whereas other people's enquiries will strike you as invasive and plain nosey. I was sometimes quite rude and short with people for no really good reason. Don't be too hard on yourself, your reaction may just be an expression of the anger stage of grief. It's quite normal to transfer your resentment at having cancer into irritation with others. It's a coping mechanism.

Summary:

Not telling people sometimes allows you to regain control of the situation.
You may need time to get used to the idea first.
It is sometimes hard to admit to your kids that you are ill and frightened, however old they are.
Breast cancer is not just an illness, it can have negative implications for a woman's sexuality.
Once you do tell people life becomes easier.
Most people will be supportive and kind.

Further Information:

American Cancer Society	http://goo.gl/5tRbp7
Breast Cancer Care	http:// goo.gl/3385N5
Health.com	http://goo.gl/c5OQzx

Chapter 10

Biopsy results: what do they mean?

If, after your first visit to the Breast Unit, everything was normal, that's wonderful. I wish you continuing good health. But if they found something abnormal, you may be at the start of a life-changing experience.

What exactly happens next depends on your hospital and your individual situation. This book isn't intended to provide comprehensive information on every possibility. If you have any specific worries, then your first step should be to speak to your breast care nurse or GP, or ask to speak to your breast specialist. If you want to read around the subject and learn more about what will happen to you, there are various excellent free booklets and website information provided by groups including Breast Cancer Care and Macmillan, amongst others.

I will tell you about the tests I had, as they are quite common and you might experience them too.

After your first visit, if they took a biopsy of the lump as they did with me, you'll probably have to wait for the pathology report, which will summarise what the laboratory found.

Let me give you a mini-biology lesson — just enough for you to understand the report.

After that small piece of your breast lump has been removed, the cells will be examined in various ways. The pathologist will see whether abnormal cells are present, which may indicate cancer. If there is no cancer ... well that's great, you probably won't be that interested in any more details.

If cancer is found, the pathologist will look at the appearance and some special characteristics of the cells. This will help decide how best to treat the cancer, and will also offer some information on your long-term outlook.

Firstly, they will want to know what *type of cells* started the cancer
- Lobular carcinoma — from the breast lobules (where milk is produced).
- Ductal carcinoma — from the ducts (tubes connecting the lobules to the nipple).

Then they will give the cancer a *grade*:

- Grade 1 means the cells are only a little abnormal
- Grade 2 is somewhere in the middle
- Grade 3 means the cells are much more obviously cancer, and are dividing and multiplying more actively.

In addition there is Ductal Carcinoma in Situ (DCIS), where the cells are becoming abnormal but are still inside the ducts. They're called pre-cancerous, or non-invasive, but can turn into full-blown cancer. DCIS can be low, moderate/intermediate, or high-grade. High-grade DCIS is most like cancer.

Next the pathologist will test the cells for special receptors — which are found on the outside of a cell and which make it respond to certain chemicals:

- Hormone receptors (to the female hormones, oestrogen and/or progesterone) make a cell grow when they come into contact with these hormones. Drugs like tamoxifen or letrozole reduce the body's natural oestrogen and can be used to treat breast cancers which have these receptors on their cells.
- Some breast cancers have another receptor, with the catchy name of HER-2. Herceptin is a drug which works by attaching onto these receptors and interfering with them.

Finally the pathologist will look for evidence that the cancer is starting to invade the blood vessels or lymph channels. Lymph channels are similar to small blood vessels and form a network around the body. They contain lymph fluid and, at various points along them, there are lymph nodes — which can become swollen if they contain cancer cells (or for other, less worrying reasons, such as if they are infected).

The blood and lymph systems act like an underground train system. If the cancer cells invade them, they can travel along them to other parts of the body. You may have further tests to see whether the cancer has spread to your lymph nodes later, but if cancer is seen in the tiny blood vessels or lymph vessels in the biopsy, it gives a heads up.

So this is the sort of information your specialist will have when they receive the biopsy results. It's easy to get confused, though. You must remember that just one small piece of the tumour was examined, so if the report uses words like 'widespread cancer' it is only talking about within that small sample. It doesn't mean that cancer has become widespread in your body; there's no way they can know that from just looking at one tiny piece of tissue.

But what about that wait between finding out you might have cancer and getting the biopsy results?

My Story

A few days after the biopsy I felt a dragging sensation in my right breast. I was particularly anxious because my late mother had suffered from breast cancer the previous year. Hers became 'inflammatory' — an aggressive form. Now I was worried that the redness I'd seen on my breast was a sign of inflammatory breast cancer too.

My imagination went into overdrive. The tumour was growing as I sat, eating into my tissues, invading my body. I couldn't possibly wait until my next appointment, I could be dead by then.

I phoned Nurse Eileen.

'Hello Kathleen, dear. Yes of course I remember you. Is everything OK?'

'I've been having a lot of pain in my breast. I'm just a bit worried ...'

'I expect it's just because of the biopsy.'

She paused, she knew that I wasn't convinced.

'I tell you what, why don't you pop along to see us. Then I can take a look. Miss Gomez is back now. If anything's amiss I'll ask her to stick her head around the door too.'

Phil offered to drive me.

This time we weren't sent to the screening section, the section for the ladies not yet stamped with the 'cancer' label, the happy innocents who'd been sent along for screening by their GPs, just as I had been just a few days earlier.

'Ah yes, take a seat over there.' The receptionist indicated to her right. This waiting room was less airy, more cramped. It was the hard-core section for proven, or in my case as near as dammit proven, cancer patients. The other patients were different here, many wearing the tell-tale headscarves that indicated chemotherapy. They seemed less relaxed, less interested in the pile of magazines. We took a seat. We didn't bother with the magazines either. Phil tried to make light conversation, but talking normally was awkward in this small and silent room.

Finally Eileen walked by. She beamed when she saw me.

'Hello Kathleen, so sorry to keep you waiting. Give me just two minutes and I'll be with you.' Once again she made me feel as if, out of the thirty or so patients who were waiting, I was the only important one.

A few minutes later, she returned and ushered us into a room. She was clearly busy, but acted as if she had all the time in the world, just for me. Over the ensuing months I would meet some people who would strongly impress me by their dedication and untiring willingness to go that extra mile for every single patient, every single day, and Eileen was one of those people.

'OK let's take a look. We'll go into this little side-room. Can you pop your top off and undo your bra, dear. Are you OK sitting there?' she called back to Phil.

She examined me as I lay on the narrow couch.

'It looks fine to me – just a bit of bruising from the biopsy – but just to be on the safe side I'll get Miss Gomez to pop in.' She placed a blue gown over me and left the room, returning a few minutes later with a smart, attractive lady in her early sixties. The lady wore a beautiful tailored, figure-hugging dress in beige wool. Her blond hair was drawn into a casual bun. She seemed aloof, but I noticed that she had kind eyes and a confident manner.

'Kathleen, this is Miss Gomez. I'll leave you with her. I'm going to pop and see if your biopsy results are ready yet. It'll be nice to get them early if they are.'

'Eileen tells me you've been having some pain after the biopsy. Let me have a look. I'm afraid my hands are cold,' she added.

She examined my breast with cool long fingers. She appeared thoughtful. I didn't understand why at the time.

48

*After what seemed a very long time, she straightened and looked at me.
'The pain is nothing to worry about. It's probably from the biopsy'.
The door opened quietly and Eileen crept in.
'I'm sorry Kathleen. The report isn't ready yet.'
'Well, thanks for trying, Eileen.'
'So when are you coming back to clinic?' Miss Gomez's question was directed at
me, but her eyes strayed to Eileen for the response.
'She's here a week on Monday, at your morning clinic.'
'Ah yes, no clinic next week. Bank holiday.' She grimaced. 'OK, we'll see you
then.'
I dressed and walked back into the main consulting room. Phil looked up as I
returned, his eyes interrogating me.
'It's all fine, I can go home now.' I tried to signal reassurance across the room
to him.
As we left, I noticed Miss Gomez staring at me. What was she thinking?*

*On the day of my next appointment, the hospital car park was full, so we had to
park on a nearby street. We'd set off in plenty of time, but ended up sprinting to
make my appointment.
We needn't have bothered. As we burst through the doors, we nearly knocked
over a large white board, on which the message 'Clinic running 90 minutes late'
was scrawled in green marker pen. In fact I wasn't seen for another two and a half
hours. I didn't mind. I was grateful to be seen, and I could hardly get annoyed
with the hard-working staff for over-running.
One can only maintain a state of acute anxiety for so long, and then boredom
neutralizes even the most serious situation. It was a lovely hot spring day, so
we sat on a bench outside to wait. Phil kept up a constant stream of silly jokes,
which made me laugh despite myself, and we read magazines and newspapers
and drank coffee.
I noticed the Italian couple from my first visit. They were sitting in a corner of
the waiting room. They didn't see me — or perhaps they did but didn't feel like
talking. She would receive her results today too. They had two young children
and she had multiple sclerosis. I prayed she wouldn't have to deal with breast
cancer too.
We waited and waited. Eventually we abandoned the sunshine and went
back inside. We didn't want to miss the appointment. As the pile of notes on*

the receptionist's desk shrank, I started to feel anxious again. Despite myself, my breathing quickened, my throat tightened and I could feel my heart beating faster than nature intended. Was I going to live or die? Was I going to have a simple lump removal or my complete breast amputated? Would I need chemotherapy? Radiotherapy? Maybe it had all been a mistake, and it wasn't even cancer at all. Maybe I'd just jumped to a neurotic conclusion?

As I became more and more tense, Phil put down the car magazine he'd brought to read and re-commenced a stream of inane chatter. Unbelievably he got me laughing again.

Finally Eileen appeared to take us through.

Miss Gomez looked up as we entered. She had an air of serious stillness that pervaded the room. Her dark eyes, large and deep, seemed to be able to read my thoughts.

'I'm sorry you've had such a long wait. I'd like to examine you again, if I may. Please go next door, take your top things off and lie on the couch.'

She certainly didn't believe in small talk, but then her clinic was already over-running by more than two hours. Nevertheless she didn't hurry her examination. Her manicured hands gently probed and felt.

She remained silent and thoughtful.

Finally 'OK, please get dressed and then we'll talk.'

I put my bra and top back on and walked back into the consulting room after her. Phil gave me a supportive look, but I could see the worry in his eyes. I sat down next to him and felt his body tense, as he waited with his pen poised to make notes on a scrap of paper.

Miss Gomez had already returned to her desk. She gazed at me.

'We have the results of your biopsy. You have a grade 2 ductal carcinoma. This means it's moderately invasive. Not the best, but not the worst type either. It's highly sensitive to oestrogen and progesterone, which is good news.'

She stared at me. She seemed to be trying to assess my reaction. Had I understood the news? Was I about to fall apart? Scream? Cry? Or just sit quietly, calm, expressionless, hiding behind a brave face? I expect she'd seen it all, over the years in this job.

I went for the brave face option.

She continued, 'When I examined you the other week the lump felt quite large.' Once more she paused, her dark eyes searching mine.

'I wanted to examine you again today to be sure. The lump is definitely quite

large, it's actually occupying about a quarter of your breast. Also, I think there may be a lump in your left breast too.'

Her delivery had been emotionless, business-like and factual, and her face was impassive, but her eyes were a talking book. I felt Phil shiver by my side.

I was completely taken aback. I seemed to have lost the use of my arms, my speech. A huge stone was sinking though my chest into my stomach, weighing me down, preventing me from coming up for air. This wasn't what I'd been expecting. I hadn't even felt any lumps, dammit. Nor had my GP, nor had the registrar I'd seen on my first visit. So why was she telling me that I had a large tumour there? On the mammogram it had only been a couple of centimetres across.

And then there was my other breast. There hadn't been any problem with my left side. She was saying that I had cancer in both breasts, and that it was huge. Thank Goodness Phil was here. I hadn't expected this turn of events. I don't think I could have coped on my own this time.

All the time my mind was racing, she was staring at me with quiet intensity. Eventually I broke the silence.

'So what happens now?'

'I want you to have an MRI scan of both breasts. We'll see you in the clinic next week to discuss the results.'

Her reply was softly spoken and final. Her face remained motionless, but her eyes betrayed her worry. It seemed obvious that she was anticipating more bad news for the next appointment.

I was panicking now. Nothing for another week? When were they going to whip out these huge tumours? I could see she needed to do the MRI, but why the delay? I thought again of my mother's aggressive breast cancer.

'I didn't feel a lump, you know. I just noticed that the skin was sometimes red, flushed. My mother had inflammatory breast cancer last year. Do you think the redness could be the same thing in my case?'

'I couldn't see any redness on your breast. Maybe it was just a skin rash,' she replied.

She sounded weary now. I tried to explain to her that the redness wasn't there all the time now, and indeed it wasn't present today, and that it definitely wasn't a rash. But she didn't seem to be listening. I gave up. I glanced down at a list of pre-prepared questions I was clutching. Many of them seemed irrelevant now, all the questions about the operation that I had wanted to ask.

I struggled to think of more things I needed answering. I wasn't ready to leave *just yet.*

'What about Herceptin? You said the tumour was sensitive to hormones, but you didn't mention Herceptin.' I knew that this was an expensive drug. There had been a controversy about the NHS not wishing to fund this treatment and I was worried that the labs hadn't bothered to test my biopsy for these receptors.

'Those results aren't back yet. We should have them next week.'

'What'll happen after the MRI scan?'

'That depends on the results. I may be able to just remove the lump, but your breast will be a lot smaller. Until I see the MRI scan I can't be sure. You may need a mastectomy'. Once again, I saw deep sympathy and silent worry in her eyes. The consultation was brief but efficient.

I couldn't think of anything else to say. My whole life had been on hold, waiting for this appointment, the biopsy results and an operation date. Instead, there was just another wait in front of me. More endless days and interminable nights, worrying, not knowing, just waiting for the next appointment.

Eileen gently shepherded us out and took us into the 'chinz room' to pick up the pieces of our shattered emotions once again.

She tried her best to answer our questions, but there was little more information she could give us.

We sipped our tea, lost in thought.

A nurse came in and handed Eileen a slip of paper.

'Ah here we are, this is your MRI appointment. Tomorrow, 11am.'

I was deeply anxious.

Eileen read my thoughts 'Please don't worry. She's very careful. She prefers to take time at the beginning, to make sure she's doing absolutely the best thing before she starts treatment.'

I couldn't argue with this approach, but this lump was causing me constant pain now and I visualized it getting bigger and bigger. At what moment would it enter my lymphatic system? Then it would be a whole new ball game. I would definitely need chemotherapy then.

There wasn't anything left to say, so we left Eileen, no doubt to dash off to see some other newly-diagnosed patient and to make them feel like they were her only patient too.

On our way out, we passed the Italian couple. They looked relaxed. I smiled at them 'How did it go?'

'Oh, good. Yes it was all good news. How about you?'

Tears came, like unwelcome guests, as I continued to smile at them.

'Not so good,' I managed to say, my throat too tight to talk easily. Phil put a hand on my back to guide me past them.

'I'm really glad for you though. Really glad.' And I meant it.

Their faces showed a mixture of relief at their own good fortune and embarrassment and concern for my situation. There was a rift between us now. She was back over the wall again, with normal people. I'd just pitched a tent in Camp Cancer.

Summary:

The pathologist will examine the biopsy of your breast lump for:

- Cancer — is there any?
- If so, what sort? Ductal or lobular?
- How aggressive is it (Grades 1-3, 3 being the most aggressive)? DCIS is a pre-cancerous condition, not dangerous, but may progress to cancer so needs treating.
- Do the cancer cells have oestrogen or progesterone receptors, or HER-2 receptors? If so they will respond to specific drugs.
- Are there cancer cells in the blood or lymph vessels in the small biopsy sample?
- The biopsy sample doesn't represent the rest of your body.

After your biopsy, you may need more tests. This means a longer wait before your cancer is treated, but it is important to get it right.

Further Information:

Breast Cancer Care   http://goo.gl/hdDQJX
Macmillan Cancer Support   http://goo.gl/AKn7ux

Dr Susan Love's Breast Book: S M Love with K Lindsey – Da Capo

Act with Love   http://goo.gl/2Pwjo1
BreastCancer.org   http://goo.gl/rKZDy6
Understanding Breast Cancer   http://bit.ly/1OjM3p3
BreastCancer.org   http://goo.gl/rKZDy6

Macmillan Cancer Support   http://goo.gl/uXVkoK

Chapter 11

Further tests you may need

Some people need an MRI scan, as I did. A breast MRI involves lying still in a large machine for 30 minutes or so. The machines use powerful magnetic fields to generate pictures of the body's tissues. These pictures provide different information to the mammogram and ultrasound examinations—so they can fill in any information gaps for the doctor.

My Story

After we left the hospital, I looked at Phil's scribbled notes. I was surprised at how little I'd taken in. When I was a hospital doctor, I used to feel slightly irritated when patients or their relatives would complain that they hadn't been given much information, when I knew I'd spent a lot of time patiently talking them through things. Yet I'd registered less than half of what Miss Gomez had told me, and I was medically trained. This whole experience was giving me new insights.

The next day Phil picked me up and drove me to the MRI scan.

'Do you have a referral form?' asked the bored-looking young girl on the reception desk.

'No. The Breast Unit arranged the scan yesterday—they didn't give me a form.'

A flicker of realisation crossed the girl's face. Her attitude changed.

'That's fine—sit down there and we'll call you in shortly.'

Soon a radiographer came out and called my name. I followed her into the scanning area, leaving Phil in the waiting room. She led me to a small curtained cubicle.

'Strip to your waist for me. Make sure you remove any metal objects—you can

lock them in this cupboard. Then put on one of those blue gowns. I'll come and get you when you're ready.'

I would go through perhaps forty or more of these gowns over the next few months. Sometimes I had to put them on with the opening at the front, sometimes at the back. Sometimes I had to put it on one way, then later I would have to switch it around. It all seemed slightly pointless, as at some point during whatever procedure I went through, the gown would inevitably be undone and my chest would be exposed to everyone in the room. I couldn't help thinking it made for a lot of unnecessary laundering. Anyway, on this occasion the gown was to open down the front.

I came out of the cubicle, so the radiographer would know I was ready. As I waited, the previous patient came out. She was in a wheelchair. A bag of clear fluid hung from the metal drip-stand attached to her wheelchair and a thin tube carried its contents to her arm. She had the tell-tale bald head and absent eyebrows and lashes of someone who'd recently had chemotherapy. She looked pale and unwell. She seemed old, but maybe it was just the ravages of the chemo. An unsmiling younger man was with her—her son, perhaps. I'm ashamed to admit that I recoiled from her appearance. I still couldn't adjust to the fact that I was now 'one of them'; a cancer patient.

The radiographer saw me and led me into the scanning room.

The MRI scan was a slightly gymnastic event. Once on the table, blue gown undone, I had to roll over onto my hands and knees and then lower my breasts into two holes in the table.

I do realise that these holes had to be large enough to accommodate all-comers—from Katie Price to Kate Moss—but as I complained later to Phil, they were huge. My bust was not particularly small, but for the first time in my life I felt rather inadequate.

'Well done. You're fairly agile. Now I need to inject some dye which will show up on the scan. I'm just going to pop this tourniquet on your arm, Can you make a fist for me?'

As the radiographer inserted the needle into the vein on the back of my hand I winced. That had really hurt. I was shocked at my own cowardice. I was going to have to toughen up; I'd be going through a lot worse than a scratch on my hand before this was over and I couldn't afford to be such a wimp. I started to panic. Was I going to be able to deal with all the pain? I was developing a new respect for the patients I'd treated in the past.

'OK, I'm just going to connect you up to this dye. It'll drip into your vein during the scan and go through your blood stream to your breasts, so we get better pictures. Here are some headphones. We won't be in the room while the scan is taking place, but we can talk to you through the headphones, and we can see you all the time.

'I need you to stay very, very still during the scan. It'll be really noisy, but I'll find some nice music to play through the headphones. What sort of music do you like?' she asked.

'I like Madonna, but anything'll be fine.'

The radiographer left the room and I lay still as my couch glided slowly into the MRI machine. The scanner started to make noisy clunking sounds and then loud, deep, repetitive vibrating noises, as if I'd accidentally lain on top of a pneumatic drill. It was a strange and unsettling sensation. Somehow those low vibrations had an uncomfortable effect, deep inside. I waited for the music to start, but it never did. I suppose she forgot. After thirty minutes or so the machine went quiet, and the radiographer came back into the room.

'All finished. You can get dressed and go. Let me just take the cannula out of your vein.'

I dragged on my clothes and went to find Phil.

A week later we were sitting in the outpatients yet again—another long wait. I hadn't slept well. I couldn't relax. I'd already read all the magazines last time. There were no new ones. Even Phil was struggling to think of amusing stories to distract me with. Our relationship seemed to be evolving into a definite friendship and I was very thankful for his support.

Much of the time we sat there we felt bored, to be honest, but every now and then the reality of my situation would bubble through and I would have a panic attack. My breathing quickened, my throat tightened and I just felt so hopeless. I was so scared—I didn't want to die. Why did I have to wait and wait interminably, just to get the damn MRI results?

Four hours late, the nurse finally called us, but she only took us to another, quieter waiting area around the corner. It was a further ten minutes before we were called in to see Miss Gomez, and, most importantly, to find out when she had scheduled my operation.

She looked more relaxed as she greeted us. Eileen was sitting quietly in the corner.

'OK. I know you've been waiting for the results so I won't waste time. The tumour in your right breast is 6 cm in diameter, so, as I thought, it's a lot bigger than it appeared on the mammogram.' She paused and looked at my reaction with those quiet brown eyes.

'The left breast is clear, though. That's really good news.' A half-smile almost broke through her trademark solemn stare.

'I'm going to ask our radiologist to take a series of biopsies of the tumour under X-ray control, so we can see how much is invasive cancer, and how much is DCIS. If some of the tumour is DCIS it's good news.'

I was bewildered. Once again, this wasn't the conversation I had expected. The previous biopsy had shown grade 2 invasive cancer. Why was she now talking about DCIS, which was a much less serious pre-cancerous condition? I was too confused to ask why DCIS was coming up now, for the first time. Instead I asked a different question, 'Do you have the HER-2 receptor results?'

'Yes, they were negative, so Herceptin isn't an option for you, unfortunately. That's often the way.' She gave me a wry smile.

'Well, if you don't have any more questions, we'll see you next week in the clinic with the biopsy results.'

Her last words went through the fog of my confusion like a bullet. Another week's delay? Doesn't she understand that this tumour is growing in me? I'd had four weeks of tests and still no arrangements had been made for the operation. Why couldn't she just get on and take the tumour out and stop wasting time?

We left the consulting room with Eileen. By now we knew our own way to the room with the chintz furniture. She made us the usual tea and biscuits, then after helping us pick up the pieces of our shattered nerves once again, she went to arrange the biopsies with the radiology department.

While she was gone Phil and I tried to make sense of what we'd just been told. A week ago the news was bad. The tumour was huge, and possibly both breasts were affected. Today Miss Gomez had seemed more optimistic, but we weren't really sure why. Yes, only one breast was affected, which was good, but the tumour on the right was now confirmed to be large. Today she'd mentioned DCIS. The outlook for DCIS was much better than for invasive cancer. I knew that. What I didn't really understand was what had changed?

Eileen came back with the tea. 'I've arranged the biopsies for you. Miss Gomez asked me to get Dr Crystal to do them. She's the best. Don't worry, we're getting closer to knowing what's going on. Miss Gomez is very thorough. You're in good

hands.' She smiled.
We drank our tea and left, drained, confused, and numb.

In fact the hospital were acting quickly. They'd done the MRI scan a day after it had been requested, and they'd arranged to do the further biopsies within the week, so the results would be ready by Miss Gomez's next clinic. But to me, with this thing growing inside me, threatening to spread around my body any minute, every delay was devastating.

This was my perception, but in fact cancer doesn't necessarily spread that quickly, and it's important to take time to find out as much about the cancer as possible before deciding on the course of treatment. The treatments are different depending on the type of cancer, how big it is, and whether it has spread. My doctor head knew that, but my woman head was not convinced. She just wanted it gone.

Some patients have different additional tests at this stage—generally with the same objective, that of assessing exactly how advanced the cancer is and what is the *stage* of the cancer.

The tumour *grade*, as discussed earlier, is based on the appearance of the cells under a microscope.

The *stage* is about the bigger picture.

A standard classification called TNM (tumour, nodes and metastasis) is used for all types of cancer. The TNM Staging system goes from Stages 1 to 4. There is a stage each for the tumour (T), the lymph nodes (N) and metastasis (M). Here's a brief explanation of these different stages:

Tumour Staging (T)
Stage T0: (or Tis): Carcinoma-in-situ (not quite cancer yet).
Stage T1: tumour is small (2cm in diameter or less) and hasn't spread to the lymph nodes.
Stage T2: the lump is larger (2 to 5cm) and/or has spread to nearby lymph nodes.
Stage T3: it is larger than 5cm.
Stage T4: the cancer has spread locally, beyond the breast, e.g. to the chest wall or the skin. This includes a special type called inflammatory cancer.

Lymph node Staging (N)
Stage N0: no lymph nodes are affected
Stage N1: means that only the armpit lymph nodes, on the same side as the tumour, have some cancer cells.
Stage N2 and N3: more lymph nodes are involved, or the lymph nodes have become matted and stuck down.

Metastasis (M)
Metastasis, or metastatic disease, means that the cancer has spread (usually through the blood or lymph vessels) to other completely different parts of the body, such as the lungs or bones.
Stage M0: the cancer hasn't spread.
Stage M1: means it has spread.

My Story

Three days later I was back in the Breast Unit. I looked around the main waiting room with a different eye. I was a seasoned patient now, and I understood the system. I recognized the women who were just coming for screening—some anxious, some relaxed and confident. Each one was living on their own personal island. There were very few interactions. The anxious patients didn't feel like talking (I knew how they felt). The patients who were just expecting a routine screening visit didn't want to talk either—their minds were elsewhere; what they would do when they left—supermarket? School pickup? Hot date? The mini ecosphere of this breast cancer department was of no real consequence to them.

I was called in to the X-ray room to see the radiologist, a bubbly petite doctor with auburn hair. She didn't look old enough to be a consultant, but then policemen have started to look ridiculously infantile too.

A nurse and radiographer were helping. As usual, we went through the blue gown ritual – this time the gown had to open down the back.

'Hello, I'm Dr Crystal. Come and sit here and we can look at your MRI scan together.' Her smile was friendly.

'This is the tumour in your right breast. You can see that it looks bigger than on the mammogram, but most of it looks like DCIS.'

'Are you saying that DCIS has a typical appearance on MRI scans?' I asked.

'Yes, exactly, but we need to take biopsies from different parts of the tumour to

confirm for definite which parts are invasive and which parts are DCIS.'

Now, at last, I started to understand. Someone had turned the lights on. My tense shoulders relaxed, as I realised that there really was a shaft of hope appearing like a sunbeam from behind the black clouds of confusing information and ominous possibilities. Miss Gomez had correctly diagnosed that I had quite a large tumour, and the original biopsy showed grade 2 cancer, so definitely some of it was invasive cancer. But the MRI scan suggested that at least some of it may be DCIS, a pre-cancerous condition. If this was true, then my outlook was much, much better. This next test would tell us for sure if this was the case.

'Come and lie down for me.' The radiographer broke into my thoughts.

Dr Crystal stayed where she was, reading my notes. The nurse was looking over her shoulder at my notes too, as the radiographer helped me onto the table.

'What's your name and date of birth?' The nurse still had her back to me. After an embarrassing silence, I deduced that she was waiting for me to respond.

'Oh I'm sorry, I thought you were talking to the doctor.' I blundered on, 'But of course you already know her name.'

'Yes she does, and I'm certainly not telling any of you my date of birth.' The doctor grimaced, as she got up and walked over to the couch, where I was lying now, under a large X-ray machine.

'First I'm going to numb your breast, and then take … maybe seven samples of the tumour. You're going to have to lie still for quite a while, but it shouldn't be painful. Do let us know if you're uncomfortable at all.'

She spoke gently and sympathetically. Although I wasn't looking forward to the multiple stabbing, she inspired confidence. I knew Miss Gomez had specifically asked for her, and Eileen had said she was the best.

The three of them started rolling me over, and manoeuvering me until I was balanced on my left side, with my right breast clamped by the plates of the X-Ray machine. Using the X-rays to guide her, Dr Crystal stuck a large needle repeatedly into my breast in different places. Each time she took a small sample of the tumour, she handed it to the nurse, who carefully placed it in a small pot, and wrote on the label exactly where the sample had been taken from.

I was fascinated. Not only did they check they had samples from the correct places using the X-ray screening, but they even X-rayed the small biopsy samples of tissue, to check they had taken biopsies containing the flecks of calcium, which they could see on the X-ray.

They were all kind—they kept checking I was warm enough, and that I was *not about to roll onto the floor, (unlikely, as I was firmly pinned to the machine by my breast), and that I was not in pain. But having your right boob squashed in an X-ray machine while a needle is repeatedly plunged into it was not my idea of how to spend an enjoyable hour or so—particularly as I literally had a front row view of the whole procedure and it wasn't for the squeamish. I was luckier than many, though. I understood what they were doing, and what all their roles were in the process, and this did make it easier to stay calm.*

Self-preservation told me that my best strategy would be to make it as easy as possible for them, so that they could relax and do the best job of taking the samples. If I complained or seemed distressed, I was worried that they might hurry the process, or not probe as thoroughly for the biopsies as they would like. So I kept quiet and stayed calm as each biopsy was taken. I uttered my usual mantra 'I'm fine' whenever asked. The staff commented on what an amazing patient I was. No, I wasn't amazing, but inside knowledge can be useful.

Summary:

After your diagnosis, you may need more tests before the doctor can start to treat you.

These tests are important, in order to make sure you are given the best, most appropriate treatment.

The delay is distressing, and the hospital should do further tests as quickly as possible.

One further test is an MRI scan, which uses strong magnetic fields to create images of the inside of your body to provide additional information to mammograms and ultrasounds—for example, it can help distinguish DCIS from invasive cancer.

They may need to take more biopsies—carefully documenting what part of your breast each sample came from, using X-ray screening. It isn't fun, but it isn't too unpleasant either, just a bit uncomfortable.

A Staging system called TNM helps to define your cancer, and helps the doctors decide on your outlook, and what treatment would be best for you. The stages are 0 up to 4, with 4 being the worst. The staging relates to the tumour itself (T), whether lymph nodes are involved (N) and whether there is spread elsewhere in the body (M).

Further Information:

Cancer.net	http://goo.gl/uqZjKU
Understanding Breast Cancer	http://bit.ly/1OjM3p3
NHS Choices	http://bit.ly/1SNOCka
Macmillan Cancer Support	http://goo.gl/uXVkoK
Cancer Research UK	http://goo.gl/yjL5pg

Chapter 12

What does knowing you have cancer feel like long-term?

I've already talked about my initial reaction—which was a mixture of shock and denial. I had to wait several months before I eventually had surgery. This was a strange limbo time. Nothing positive was happening, I was just waiting, harbouring the knowledge that the tumour was inside me, an alien, growing bigger, free to run riot through my vulnerable body in any way it chose, or so it seemed. I will try to share some of my emotional experiences during that time and beyond.

My Story

The ensuing weeks and months were an emotional roller-coaster.

Looking back, I was mainly in denial. There were certainly dark times. Would I die? If so, how soon? I experienced moments of fear, and, sometimes acute panic. But most of the time, I was encased in a strange euphoria. My senses seemed to be heightened—and colours were more intense. I was very conscious of nature. I became extremely observant, acutely aware of the tiniest object. I noticed the delicate features on the smallest insect, the rainbow reflections on the tiny wings, the graceful movement of its head; the wonderful perfume of a flower. The world just seemed so beautiful. Maybe I was trying to experience as much as possible, because my time might suddenly be much less than I'd anticipated, maybe it was just a state of shock? I don't know, but it was noticeable.

Coupled with this, I felt a bit of a fraud. Everyone who'd heard my news was devastated. Some put me on a pedestal as a heroine, some as a martyr, and yet it seemed there was nothing wrong with me. I felt and looked fit and well. Yes, there was this small bit of cancer, but as soon as she had the pathology results, the nice surgeon was going to remove it all, and everything was going to be fine. So I didn't really deserve all the fuss and sympathy. It wasn't as if I had proper cancer, not like some poor souls.

And then I began to feel 'special'. I had CANCER (a bit like having a platinum card).

'I'm sorry, I have cancer, I really can't queue up with everyone else, could you see me right away?'

'I have breast cancer, how about giving me your seat?'

'How dare you shout at me? Don't you know I have cancer?'

In truth, I only used this trump card a couple of times, and each time I did I felt guilty using such a lever, even when I felt pretty awful during the radiotherapy, but when I did, the effect was powerful. The one simple word "Cancer" opens an encyclopaedia of thoughts, feelings, associations, memories, and fears in everyone's mind—and no one is immune.

Sometimes denial switched to anger. I would like to apologise to all the sweet old ladies who I glared at, wondering what exactly they had contributed to the world which gave them the right to have achieved a ripe old age?

I also felt angry at some of the responses I encountered when I told people my news, such as:

'Don't worry you're going to be fine! I have a friend and she had the same thing as you and she's cured now.'

Really? Oh good, I'll tell the hospital not to bother with all the expensive tests they'd planned, because, somehow, you know the size, histological grade and receptor-status of my tumour, and whether or not my lymph nodes are invaded. Not only that, but miraculously you also know of a reference case with exactly the same characteristics as my disease, so you can accurately predict my prognosis.

'Oh yes, I've had loads of breast lumps! No problem, they just whip them out – a piece of cake!'

And were any of them cancer?

'No'

Well that isn't quite the same then, is it?

And probably the worst response, whilst I was waiting unexpectedly long for my surgery:

'Oh a friend has just had her operation for breast cancer. She had it done within a couple of weeks.'

'But I'm having to wait months for mine.'
'Ah yes, but hers was serious.'

Sometimes people are as shocked as you are, and accidently say the wrong thing. Sometimes they don't think, and sometimes, maybe, they are not the sort of friends you really need. However, my reaction to their comments, and my perception of what they said, reflected my emotional state too. So be a little circumspect before you sever a friendship. Your friends and loved ones may be hurt by your unexpected retorts to something they have said, and it could help them to understand that your reaction is not 'personal', just a human reaction to an impossible situation.

I found the most helpful response to my news was an acknowledgement of the seriousness of my condition.

My Story

My emotions were supercharged for a very long period of time. Eventually, after the operation, and all the radiotherapy, time did its job and they gradually stopped bouncing off the ceiling like rubberized grenades, exploding intermittently with no warning.

My reaction, unsurprisingly, was related to possible death. Yes, I was worried about my appearance and womanhood and so on, but underneath this was a real fear of imminent death. This is most people's deepest fear. At first it was just too awful to consider. The sudden change from perfectly healthy with the prospect of a long and boring future, to I've got cancer and don't know if I'll be around next year, was just too enormous for me to handle. It was too unbelievably painful to think about for very long, but the thought would frequently barge into my consciousness. I'd awake in the morning, feeling fine, then suddenly I'd remember, and the cold sweat and nausea would kick in. My two kids were the most important things in my life. I couldn't bear the thought of not being around for them. I couldn't bear their pain of losing a parent when they were only young adults themselves.

I started to consider more practical implications too. I'd always worked hard, and I'd been fairly frugal. I'd managed to save a little nest-egg. I'd imagined it would keep me secure in my old age, and then it would give me great pleasure to pass on what was left to my children when I departed this life. It pained me that now a large chunk would go in inheritance tax. I may not have time to spend any of it. This was never my wish. All those long hours I'd worked—for what?

Human beings are capable of adjusting to pretty much anything, though. As I got used to the idea, the sweats and the nausea eased and I began to think more calmly. I always knew I was going to die sometime. I didn't believe that death was the end. OK, I wasn't expecting to go so soon, but I wasn't the first and I wouldn't be the last.

This is what Kübler-Ross calls acceptance. Once I accepted death, there was nothing else that could hurt me. Even though the tests later showed that my outlook was much better than originally predicted, my attitude towards death and life has been permanently changed by this experience of uncertainty. I now really do appreciate every single day of my life. I try not to take it for granted, or wish my time away. I am also aware that there are far worse diseases to have than cancer, or at least some cancers. None of us know when that guy with the long black dress and scythe will pop by. Once we accept this, we can find ourselves curiously liberated. This may sound weird, but in some ways I feel privileged to have lived through cancer—it taught me things that I probably couldn't have learned any other way.

But even apart from death, cancer can have other devastating psychological effects. Ignorant of the amazing reconstructive surgery options, I was initially convinced that my breasts would be mutilated. I assumed that I would no longer be attractive as a woman. I found this extremely difficult to cope with; I wasn't ready to be written off as a sexual being. I was reticent to even let men know I had breast cancer, in case they visualized me without a breast.

Having endured the treatment and emerged successfully, my attitude and confidence level has changed. Because I'm lucky to live in a first world country, I had access to highly technical diagnostic machines which were able to assess my cancer with great accuracy. This meant that my treatment could be individually planned to maximise benefit and minimise side-effects. Every woman in the UK also has access to sophisticated surgery (provided there is no medical reason against it), meaning that their breasts can end up looking as good as they did before the breast cancer surgery.

But at the time I didn't know that, and I wasn't in a mental state to go and find out. In retrospect, one of the reasons for my anxiety was the progressively worse news I had received during the earlier appointments, when every visit seemed to unpeel another layer of problems. It seemed that my cancer was becoming more serious with each new revelation. I concluded that I was highly likely to die—and soon.

However, I had not asked the medical staff that vital question: 'Am I going to die of this cancer, and if so when?'

Why didn't I ask it? After all it is the key question associated with a cancer diagnosis, isn't it? Partly I didn't ask because I knew they wouldn't be able to say for certain until they had all the test results.

This highlights a quandary that exists within the current UK medical system. There is a culture of not giving a patient false hope. However, as a patient, I noticed that this often translated into an unnecessarily gloomy impression. Often there are so many caveats, even with every positive statement, that the patient can make an unnecessarily pessimistic interpretation of what doctors and nurses tell them.

I can understand that staff couldn't give me accurate information until they knew my exact cancer stage and type. If they'd tried to discuss the large number of potential outcomes, some of which would turn out to be not relevant for me, they could have worried me unnecessarily. Except…not really. Of course I was going to wonder about the worst case scenario, and I was more than capable of imagining my own list of potential outcomes over the course of what ended up being several weeks of tests.

If I'd said at the outset that I thought it likely my death was imminent, they would probably have offered me some cautious reassurance. If you have similar dark thoughts, I would advise you to share them with the doctor or nurse—you might be pleasantly surprised by their response, and if not, well at least you're a bit clearer about your concern.

These were my thoughts and experiences. There is much more which I have not dwelt on, but help is available if you are troubled with different aspects of living with cancer, either your own or that of someone close to you. You might want to know how it can affect your relationship with a partner, how to deal with the symptoms of stress which are frequently associated with it for example. Val Sampson and Debbie Fenlon have written an excellent book which deal with many of these issues.

Summary:

Other people react in different ways to hearing someone has cancer—some people say the wrong thing for various reasons. Sometimes they are in a state of shock too, sometimes they just don't understand.

Treatment of Breast cancer has changed dramatically over recent years in the first world—not only maximising anti-cancer treatment, but minimising side-effects and optimising cosmetic appearance of the breasts.

Further Information:

Book: The Breast Cancer Book by V. Sampson & D Fenlon. Vermilion, 2000

Chapter 13

Breast cancer treatment

Once all your tests are completed, your doctor will discuss with you what treatment you need. Depending on your particular case, they may recommend some or all of the following: surgical operation(s), medication, radiotherapy. Research is ongoing all the time, and breast cancer treatment information becomes outdated almost as soon as it's written—therefore it's useful to use reputable internet sites to check on latest treatments. However below is an overview of some of the treatments you may need to know about.

Surgery
It may be possible to just remove the lump by itself (a lumpectomy or wide local excision). If it's a large lump, your surgeon may need to refashion your breast, and possibly reduce the size of your other breast to match. Alternatively, for various reasons, your doctor may recommend a mastectomy (where the whole breast is removed).

If you do need a mastectomy, your breast can sometimes be rebuilt (a reconstruction) during the same operation. This means that you wake up with two breasts. Sometimes, for medical reasons, it needs to be done later, and you'll be left with an absent breast for a period of time. In this case you can use an artificial breast (prosthesis) inside your bra. You can usually have a reconstruction later, if you want.

There are various surgical techniques used to reconstruct a breast after it has been removed. An implant of artificial material such as silicone can be inserted, or a new breast can be fashioned from your own body tissue, such as muscle from your back, or muscle/fat from your belly. There are advantages and disadvantages to all these approaches and your surgeon should discuss these with you to help you decide.

Often the operation is done first, followed by other treatments. However sometimes other treatments may be given before surgery, to shrink the tumour (neo-adjuvant therapy).

Because most breast cancers start in the breast ducts, which pass through the nipple, your nipple will usually have to be removed to make sure no cancer cells are left behind. There are some clever ways to 'replace' the nipple, such as using skin tattoos, or by 'making' a new nipple from another part of your body, or by using the surface skin of your own nipple once the ducts have been carefully removed. You can even get 'stick-on' nipples. These options don't sound too great (I didn't think so anyway) but they are actually surprisingly good, and the tattoos look quite realistic. Again you should be offered a choice about this.

Your surgeon will usually remove some lymph nodes during the operation. He may just remove a couple, to test whether the cancer has spread there (called a sentinel node biopsy), or he may need to remove more. Sometimes when lymph nodes are removed from your armpit, your arm will swell, permanently (lymphoedema), so the surgeon will only remove extra lymph nodes if cancer has definitely spread to them. Doctors used to remove all the armpit lymph nodes in everyone, but then research taught them that this wasn't always necessary.

Medication

For many women, just removing the cancerous lump isn't enough to stop the cancer coming back. For some women, surgery isn't an option for various reasons. Both these groups of women may need medication, either for a short time or for many years. After many careful studies, treatment regimes to cover most situations have been developed. There are various medicines which can help treat breast cancer or prevent its recurrence, and they generally fall into the following types:

Chemotherapy

Chemotherapy, also called cytotoxic therapy, refers to strong anti-cancer treatments which damage cells that are actively dividing. This means they can damage normal cells too, but they tend to damage cancer cells most.

Careful choice of dosing will facilitate the destruction of as many cancer cells as possible, whilst allowing normal cells to recover. This means that chemotherapy often has many unwanted effects too. Normal cells which also divide frequently, such as the cells of our gut, tend to be affected most, so diarrhoea and sore mouth can be a problem, amongst other things.

Chemotherapy drugs differ in their effectiveness against different cancers, and in terms of how toxic they are to non-cancer cells. A great deal of research has led to the development of regimes which aim to use the most effective drugs for your particular cancer and to give them in the best amounts and at the most effective frequencies. These regimes are modified as new information becomes available, and thus can change over time. Websites such as Macmillan and Breast Cancer Care provide up-to-date details on current regimes. Chemotherapy may be offered for different reasons. A common reason is if the cancer has already spread outside the breast, for example to the lymph nodes. A course of chemotherapy for breast cancer typically involves several bouts over four to six months—but again this will depend on your particular circumstances.

Hormone Treatments

Many breast tumours have special receptors which mean they can be stimulated to grow by female hormones—oestrogen and progesterone. The laboratory will test your tumour cells for these. If present, drugs such as tamoxifen or aromatase inhibitors such as letrozole, anastrozole and exemestane can be useful. They interfere with your natural oestrogens and can reduce the risk of the cancer returning. Long-term studies are providing more and more information on the benefits of these drugs, and they seem to have a protective effect for years after the first cancer treatment. Generally tamoxifen is used in pre-menopausal women, who can then switch to an aromatase inhibitor after the menopause. But even this is changing as more information becomes available from recent large-scale studies.

Targeted Therapies (including Herceptin)

Targeted therapies are designed to attack just the cancer cells, and not your normal cells. Some breast cancer cells have a large number of HER-2 receptors. Herceptin (also called trastuzumab) is a drug which binds to these receptors and stops the cells growing or dividing. It also helps your body's own immune system destroy the cancer cell. As normal cells don't have so many HER-2 receptors, Herceptin preferentially attacks cancer cells. The labs will test your tumour for these receptors to assess whether you will benefit from Herceptin. It is useful but does have some undesirable side-effects, including heart problems.

Radiotherapy

You may or may not require radiotherapy. If you do, you will usually have it after your surgery and/or chemotherapy. It is generally given as powerful X-ray treatment, which is capable of destroying cancer cells. Sometimes other methods are used, such as implanting radio-active isotopes into the area of a tumour, or into the tumour itself. These isotopes emit radioactive waves, giving ongoing treatment to the local area for so long as they are left in the body. At the time of writing these are not usually used for breast cancer, although there have been some studies to see how well they may work.

Radiotherapy is most effective on cells which are actively dividing, which is why they tend to kill cancer cells more than normal cells. However they can damage normal cells too. The part of the body treated with X-rays is carefully planned so that as much of the cancer as possible is dosed by the X-rays, while as little normal tissue as possible is included in the radiation beam. For example, a beam of X-rays may be directed at the tumour from two or more different directions, so that the tumour itself gets at least double the dose, whilst any normal tissues that get in the way will only get a single dose.

If the lymph nodes under your arm were found to contain cancer, then these and other lymph nodes around the breast may be treated with radiotherapy at the same time.

The length of treatment will vary, and is changing over time as more information becomes available, but three weeks (Monday to Friday) of daily treatment followed by a week of boost treatment (more localized just to the site of the cancer) is typical.

Experimental treatment and Drug trials

You may also be offered experimental treatment or asked whether you want to take part in a clinical trial. Some clinical trials study very new drugs that have not yet been approved by the regulatory authorities, so more information is still needed on their safety and beneficial effects. Other studies look at treatments which are already in use, but investigate different ways of giving the treatment (for example more or less frequently, or for longer or shorter periods), to see if benefit or side-effects can be improved.

There are many considerations and there are many advantages in taking part in some clinical trials, but there should be no moral pressure on you to take part, and if you do agree, you can withdraw at any time, without giving a reason, and you will be given the same care and treatment opportunities regardless. The advantages of taking part in a trial with a new (unapproved) drug mean that you may have access to an effective treatment before it is available for doctors to use by any other means. If you have a serious and life-threatening cancer, this may be a good option. The disadvantages are that less is known about the drug than more established therapies, including how well it really works, and how safe it is. The overall risk-benefit balance will depend very much on your particular situation, and you should be able to discuss this carefully with the staff who are conducting the trial.

So these are the possible treatments you may be offered. I'd had all the tests I needed, my surgeon now knew what sort of cancer I had, how big it was, exactly where it was, and that the other breast was clear. So what treatment would she recommend?

My Story

Another week on, and I was sitting with Phil in the out-patient department once again.

So far, I'd had a mammogram, a single biopsy, an MRI scan and seven more biopsies. Now, surely there could be no more reasons not to just get on and remove the tumour, before it grew to the size of a football?

I even had a small overnight bag with me in case they decided to admit me for my operation straight away. We waited the statutory two to three hours before being called in.

Miss Gomez was smart and cool as always—another tailored dress, cut just above the knee, with a square neckline, this time in dark blue. Eileen wore matching baby blue dress with grey cardigan (and no, I'm sure they didn't colour-coordinate their clothes deliberately).

As we waited for the verdict, I felt Phil's arm against me, stiff and tense, as was mine. Miss Gomez seemed to take ages before she spoke.

'Quite good news. Most of the biopsies showed DCIS'. As usual, she paused and looked at me.

Straining forward, I willed her to keep talking. What was the bottom line? What was she going to do? Get on with it woman, you're not announcing who got knocked out of 'Strictly Come Dancing'. This is my life, and I can't take any more suspense.

'Some of the biopsies showed grade two carcinoma, as we saw on the earlier biopsy. So, overall, it looks like you have a tumour of six centimetres in diameter, of which probably two to two and a half centimetres is grade two carcinoma. The rest is DCIS.'

She was silent again after her statement. Her dark eyes stared at me calmly, expectantly. I didn't know what she was waiting for me to say. I just wanted to know what was going to happen to me.

'So what's the plan?' I said, eventually.

She seemed pensive, 'Let me examine you again first.'

Unprompted, I walked into the adjoining examination room, stripped to the waist and lay on the narrow couch. We didn't bother with the blue gown ritual. I think we both had similar views on wasteful laundry. She seemed to examine me for ages, gently feeling and moulding my breasts with her hands.

Her thoughts were so loud it seemed as if I could hear them... 'If I remove it, there'll be quite a hole, but there should be just about enough breast tissue left. If I bring this part over, and move this bit round... yes, should be possible...'

She waited for me to dress and sit back down, next to Phil, in the consultation room.

'I can remove the tumour. It's big, so it'll mean removing a quarter of your breast. It's called a Wide Local Excision operation. The alternative is a mastectomy. Which would you prefer?'

I was confused. I didn't really know enough about the options. As usual Miss Gomez had nearly finished a very busy clinic. Maybe she had explained the various operations so many times that morning that she didn't realize she hadn't really explained them to me. Maybe she thought that as I was a doctor I should somehow know? But I knew little more than the layman about all the modern operations which are available now, and their merits.

Eventually, as she continued to stare silently at me, I tested the water,

'I suppose just removing the tumour would be best?'
My comment at least elicited a reaction.

'If we go for the wide local excision, there'll be a lot of scar tissue, and the breast will be smaller than the other one. It'll be difficult in the future to know whether any new mammography changes are due to scarring, or to a new tumour, so you may need more biopsies in the future.'

She paused before continuing. 'You'll need radiotherapy afterwards. This'll make the breast shrink even more. I'll need to wait until after all the radiotherapy to see how much shrinkage occurs, then I can reduce your other breast to match.'

She paused again, staring at me intently. I nodded to indicate I'd understood, then she continued. 'The pathologist will examine the tumour after I've removed it. If he finds that some of the tumour was left behind, I may need to go back and do a mastectomy.'

It all sounded very negative. Maybe she was trying to steer me towards mastectomy with breast reconstruction? Confused, I tried to work out what option I was supposed to go for. I never had much time for poker and I seemed to be second-guessing what cards she was holding, with infinitely high stakes.

'Oh, OK. So maybe a mastectomy with a reconstruction would be best?'

She took a breath. 'Well if that's what you want, there are different types of reconstruction. You could have an artificial implant, or there are various onco-plastic procedures I could use, such as a latissimus dorsi flap, which uses muscle and fat from behind your shoulder to replace the breast tissue. Alternatively, fat can be taken from your tummy to replace the breast tissue. This is called a DIEP flap. It stands for Deep Inferior Epigastric Perforator, which refers to the blood vessel involved. You probably wouldn't need radiotherapy if you had a mastectomy.'

She looked at me expectantly. She didn't exactly glance at her watch, but I was conscious that her clinic should have finished hours ago, and she was already very late for wherever she should be right now. I'd been in the same situation myself as a hospital doctor, so I knew how she felt. But my brain felt numb. She seemed to be asking me to make a critical decision in a few minutes and I didn't even feel capable of deciding whether I wanted a cappuccino or an espresso. I glanced at Phil. He was scribbling notes feverishly but looked as bewildered and distressed as I felt.

I tried to focus. I remembered that Eileen had commented that implants usually looked strange in older women, often pointing skyward, instead of hanging pendulously like the other normal breast, so I dismissed that option. Call me vain, but I wasn't ready to put my body in the garbage bag yet. I really didn't want to look like a freak.

I was quite sporty, and loved yoga, so the physical and cosmetic effect of removing part of my latissimus dorsi muscle didn't appeal either. It sounded very lop-sided and I would be left with some weakness in the right shoulder.

However, the DIEP-flap, which involved replacing my breast tissue with fat from my tummy – now that did have an instant appeal—an NHS boob job AND a tummy tuck - maybe this cancer thing had an up-side? I could certainly spare some belly fat, and this operation should leave me with the least disfigurement too as far as I could see.

'I'd like to have the mastectomy and DIEP-flap reconstruction.' I replied, confident that I'd made a good choice.

'I can't offer that operation—you'd need to go to a plastic surgeon for that,' she replied flatly, and with an air of finality. She didn't seem to offer an explanation of how this could be achieved.

I felt nonplussed, bewildered, flat. What did she mean?

It sounded as if this wasn't a genuine option for me, after all. Maybe it was only for younger women, more deserving of a perfect body. Not someone past their sell-by date, like me?

She hadn't specifically offered to refer me to a plastic surgeon, and in any case, my over-riding fear was further delay of my life-saving surgery. This would be inevitable if I started again from what seemed like the beginning. So I dismissed the only option that had seemed appealing. It had seemed too good to be true anyway.

So what should I do? She'd painted a negative picture of the wide local excision operation, but it seemed that in practice, I only had the choice of that or a mastectomy with a reconstruction using either an artificial implant or part of my back muscle, neither of which appealed to me for cosmetic or functional reasons. To be honest, I'd not been able to bring myself to do much reading on it. I was totally reliant on what she was telling me, and the information she'd offered seemed to have more missing pieces than my kids' old jigsaws.

I felt suddenly weary. I tried to ask more questions, but her explanations were confusing—she seemed to switch from describing one procedure to another and I was finding it difficult to keep track of her thought process. It seemed that, whatever I chose, I would be left with a chest that even Gok Wan couldn't salvage.

She really didn't appear to understand how little information she'd given me, and how confusing her explanations had been. The woman was overworked and exhausted—it wasn't her fault. But it wasn't my fault either, and I needed proper guidance.

Finally I tried an approach which had worked well for me in other situations, 'If you were in my shoes, what operation would you choose?'

'But I'm not in your shoes. Only you can decide what is best for you.'

And I knew her automatic response was sincere. All patients are different, and nowadays, patient choice is encouraged. However, the doctor is the expert, and when I had worked in hospitals the doctor would decide what was best and advise accordingly without fearing his actions would be twisted and misinterpreted by a 'no win no fee' ambulance-chaser at a later date. It wasn't always right, but it wasn't always wrong either.

She carried on staring at me, waiting for a decision. I couldn't hold her up any longer, I knew she was busy, after all, she was going to be my saviour. She was the person who would remove the deadly tumour from my bosom. So I accepted her explanation and made one of the most important decisions of my life on little more than the toss of a coin.

I chose the lump removal. I crossed my fingers as I said it, hoping that her pessimistic warnings were overstated, and everything would be fine. I was desperate for the cancer to be removed without any further delays, but I felt so empty.

'OK then, that's what we'll do.' She seemed relieved that I'd decided.

'I'll take the sentinel node biopsy at the operation. Eileen will explain the logistics. Let's find a date.'

She opened a well-thumbed desk diary.

'July 6th,' she announced in an emotionless voice.

Had I heard her right?

'July? But that's nearly two months away. It's nearly three months already since I first noticed the problem, that means almost five months altogether.'

'Yes' she returned my gaze with weary eyes, 'it's outside the recommended time-frame, but it's the first slot I have.' As always, her face was impassive and her voice was deadpan, but her eyes filled the gaps. I suspected that she wasn't happy with what she was offering me, but it was genuinely the best she could do, I was sure of that.

'I tell you what, we'll start you on Tamoxifen in the meantime. Your tumour is

78

hormone-sensitive so it may help.'

Tamoxifen would block my natural oestrogens and starve the tumour. However it would also send me into menopause. Normally I wouldn't have started this drug until after my surgery and radiotherapy, but I suppose she—and I—felt the overwhelming need to be doing 'something'. So she wrote a prescription and Eileen gently ushered us out of the consulting room and back to the chintz room.

Once we were sitting down, she explained that the department was temporarily reduced to one consultant instead of three, and Miss Gomez was having to cope as best as she could alone, hence the delay.

There wasn't much else to say.

We sipped our tea and failed miserably to make small talk.

Then a nurse burst into the room,

'Oh, good, you're still here. Miss Gomez may be able to fit you in sooner—don't go for a minute.'

She dashed out of the room again.

My emotions soared, the room brightened, the chintz suite took on a new charm, the hospital-issue tea became a culinary masterpiece—there was a God after all, and I knew He wouldn't let me down.

We waited ten stomach-churning minutes until the nurse came back. She looked serious,

'I'm so sorry. She really tried but it isn't possible, so it's still July 6th.'

Phil dropped me home. He had to rush off. I fumbled in my handbag for my key, opened the door and threw the overnight bag down in the hall. I couldn't face unpacking it. It was going to be a long afternoon and another bad night. I shouted to the empty room:

'I'm so frightened. What am I going to do?'

I was numb. How could I get through the next two months knowing that the cancer was continuing to grow and invade; knowing that it could reach my lymph nodes during this waiting period, and that I would be helpless to stop it?

I phoned my kids. I knew they were anxious to hear what had happened. They were a fabulous support, and I don't know what I would have done without their love.

They couldn't remove the tumour though. It seemed no one could, at least not for a further two months.

Looking back, I'm not sure how much of my confusion was down to poor explanation and how much was my inability to process information due to shock. Maybe there was an element of both. I know Phil had taken written notes, but he was shocked too, and perception is everything—my perception, his perception, Miss Gomez' perception. We each had our personal truths, and all of them were different. I know from my time as a hospital doctor that sometimes I would carefully explain something to a patient or their relatives, yet a day later they would complain to me that no one had spoken to them at all. They weren't being difficult or stupid, they just hadn't absorbed the information. But I also believe that my consultant, who was excellent and conscientious, had an unacceptably high workload when she was treating me, and she was exhausted and rushed. This was not the NHS at its glorious best. In addition, I later discovered that Miss Gomez could have offered to refer me to a plastic surgeon capable of doing the operation I had requested—the mastectomy with reconstruction using my abdominal fat. Maybe I should have pressed for her to follow this option, but I didn't know my entitlements then and the NHS wasn't how I remembered it.

And then there was the two month delay. It's possible that Miss Gomez was doing a juggling act, trying to treat women with the most advanced, aggressive disease first, but not leaving other women too long either. But I didn't see that. All I saw was that I had breast cancer. It was invading me and could kill me if it wasn't stopped in its tracks. It was like being locked in a house with a knife-wielding maniac, and having to run from room to room, dodging him for two whole months before salvation arrived.

As an aside, Miss Gomez prescribed Tamoxifen for me. Neither the hospital nor my GP informed me that, with my cancer diagnosis, I was entitled to a medical exemption certificate—allowing me free prescriptions for five years. I found out several months later, by chance. When I asked my GP's secretary to complete the paperwork for me, she appeared embarrassed, and commented that they had assumed the hospital would have told me this. It is easy enough for such things to slip through the communication net, but cancer can prove expensive in many ways – lost working hours, hospital visits and car park fees, and prescriptions for example. As the advert says, 'Every little helps.'

Summary:

Treatment of breast cancer usually involves surgery and/or medication and/or radiotherapy

Surgery may involve just removing the lump or you may need a mastectomy, where the whole breast is removed. The breast can be reconstructed after the mastectomy.

Nearby lymph nodes may need to be removed, or treated with radiotherapy, if cancer is found in them. A sentinel biopsy can establish whether cancer has spread to them.

Usually the nipple has to be removed as well as the breast lump, but there are various clever ways of replacing it.

You may need drug treatment—either chemotherapy or hormone therapy or targeted therapy such as Herceptin, or a combination of all of these.

You may need radiotherapy too, typically a 3 week course followed by a week's booster course.

There are many clinical trials for cancer. If you are offered a chance to take part in them, think about it carefully. There are advantages and disadvantages. You are free to decide without any pressure.

Communication can be a problem when people are ill. Sometimes, for whatever reason, hospital staff do not communicate effectively. In addition, shocked patients and relatives cannot always absorb information. Steps should be taken to make sure they understand what is happening and what their options are.

If you request or need a treatment for your cancer which isn't available at your hospital, your consultant can refer you to another hospital where it is available (provided there is no medical reason why you shouldn't have the treatment).

Further Information:

Breast Cancer Care   http://goo.gl/0FdBnk

Chapter 14

What if you are unhappy with your treatment? Taking control

Although I hadn't been refused my preferred operation, I had got the impression that it wasn't a real option, and no one had made any effort to persuade me otherwise. If I'm honest, I half felt that I wasn't entitled to this operation. I knew it was complicated and took many hours, and had to be performed by a highly qualified plastic surgeon. Surely such an operation must be rationed? There could never be enough resources for every woman to have it. Wasn't this intended for young, attractive women struck down by cancer, not me? Surely a middle-aged old bat like me should just be grateful that they were removing the cancer?

So my first reaction wasn't to fight for the chance of that operation, but rather to accept what I was being offered, despite all my misgivings.

During my cancer experience, I came across some people who would unashamedly demand the best for themselves, and were not frightened of appearing belligerent or making themselves unpopular—and they usually got what they wanted. However, I believe that British people generally are not good at fighting for themselves. We tend to be self-deprecating, a facet of our character that appears in our language:

'Sorry to bother you, but ...'

'I don't want to be a nuisance ...'

'Would you mind ...?'

'I'd be very grateful if you would ...'

How many times have we used these expressions? In restaurants, shops, or on the phone, when we've received appalling service and are merely asking for what we deserved in the first place?

Where our health is concerned, many people's natural reaction is to become more submissive. We're dependent on the medical profession to save us, and we don't want to alienate any of them.

Doctors are not put on quite such a high pedestal as they used to be. When I first qualified, sweet old ladies with huge surgical scars often had no idea what operation had been performed on them. They just told me, 'The doctor said I needed it.' Things have improved for the better in this regard, and we are generally more informed about health and are not afraid to use the internet. However I think we still have a great deal to learn about asserting ourselves where medical care is concerned.

If you have a serious illness, you need to be prepared to be proactive in making sure you get the best care. At the end of the day, you will come across excellent and dedicated doctors, nurses and medical technicians, and you will also meet the occasional one who just turns up for the pay cheque. Either way, you are the one person who knows the most about you, and you are the person most consistently motivated to make sure you get the best care.

Having said all that, it is also important to remember that your doctor has many years of training and experience and might, just might, know a great deal more about your disease than you do. Sometimes people look things up on the internet and assume they know as much as the doctor. Nobody is an instant expert, and you should always listen to and consider what your doctor tells you. A balanced approach is important.

It's interesting that faced with a life-threatening illness, I felt that I should be grateful for any chance of survival the experts offered me. Any further cosmetic demands seemed almost bad taste—somehow ungrateful, shallow. Well, just in case you're tempted to think along those lines too, don't. It's true that in many countries of the world, even a basic life-saving operation would be an unattainable luxury, but in the UK, and other first world countries, we do have more options.

Naturally, your care should give you the best chance of cure. However, breasts also symbolize womanhood, and for many women, there are huge feelings of loss of femininity and attractiveness wound up in the treatment. The medical community is well aware of this, and clinical trials are testing and comparing treatment regimens all the time, to make sure that not only does a woman receive the most effective treatment for her cancer, but also that the damage to her breasts and body is minimized, and she has the best cosmetic outcome. You have every right to expect this level of treatment.

There is a body in the UK called the National Institute for Health and Care Excellence (better known as NICE). It provides guidance and recommendations on best practise in medical care for various illnesses, including breast cancer. Hospitals and general practices usually follow these guidelines. At the time of writing, there are NICE clinical guidelines for early and locally advanced breast cancer, and a separate guideline for advanced breast cancer. These guidelines summarise the care a patient should expect, and what treatments are available. Other countries may have similar documents. They are freely available on the internet, and it's worth looking at them. They give you a good overview of current treatment, and they also give you an idea of what you should expect from your care.

For example, these guidelines recommend doctors to:

'Discuss immediate breast reconstruction with all patients who are being advised to have a mastectomy, and offer it except where significant comorbidity or (the need for) adjuvant therapy[1] may preclude this option. All appropriate breast reconstruction options should be offered and discussed with patients, irrespective of whether they are all available locally.'

So not only should every woman have the option of waking up after her cancer operation with a 'normal' breast (provided there are no medical reasons against this) but, equally important, she should be offered the option of ALL suitable methods of achieving this. Although all suitable procedures were described to me, when I specifically requested one of these I was made to feel it was not readily available to me.

---

1   *adjuvant therapy is further treatment to improve survival

The guidelines also define acceptable wait periods for initial consultation and parts of the treatment, for example:

> *'Start adjuvant chemotherapy or radiotherapy as soon as clinically possible within 31 days of completion of surgery in patients with early breast cancer having these treatments.'*

Currently some centres have difficulties achieving these timelines, but if you are not offered treatment within the recommended time-frame you can challenge this.

These are just some examples of what you can expect as standard care, but the trouble is that when you receive news about cancer, you're in a poor shape to even think straight, never mind challenge the doctor. Most medical care in the UK is excellent, but you do need to question it if necessary.

If you're not happy with the treatment offered, you have various options. First, explain your concerns to your consultant, or talk to your breast care nurse. It may be that your worries are misplaced, or there is a genuine reason why a particular course of treatment has been decided on for you, but it's important that you understand this.

You may be worried that you will be regarded as a trouble-maker. In fact generally that was not my experience. I found most (although not all) of the staff sympathetic, and at the end of the day it's your body, your life. Once the damage is done, it's too late, so speak up loud and clear, and don't worry about upsetting anyone. You have to live with the decisions, and any mistakes. 'Oops, sorry!' may have life-time implications for you.

If you're getting nowhere, you can put your concerns in writing; sometimes these are taken more seriously than spoken concerns. You can go back and talk to your GP, who may be able to clarify a misunderstanding or talk to your consultant on your behalf—or they can send you to a new consultant for a second opinion.

If you're still banging your head against a medical brick wall, you can contact Patient Advice and Liaison Service (PALS). There should be a PALS officer in every hospital and also a separate officer for problems with GPs. They will sometimes intervene and help. Above all, be persistent and do not take no for an answer if you are unhappy.

There's also a formal NHS complaints procedure—but really, if you've reached that point something has gone badly wrong. Receiving good care is far more important than the hollow victory of winning a complaint after the damage has been done.

When I was diagnosed with breast cancer, Michael, my lovely yoga teacher told me,

'Own the situation Kathleen. Control it, don't let it control you.' I believe he was meaning this on a more metaphysical level, but how prophetic those words would turn out to be.

I will tell you what I did, and what I achieved, as a guide, but your problem will be different, or maybe you'll have no problems—which of course is the best option.

My Story

The lump, which I'd failed to feel just a few weeks ago, was now very definite. It ached constantly. It was always in my thoughts.

I considered my situation. When Miss Gomez gave me an operation date two months away, she'd mentioned a study which showed that a delay of less than three months from diagnosis would not affect overall survival. She was competent, caring and knowledgeable, and this statistic clearly kept her going. But I'd worked in research for nearly twenty years and I knew the pitfalls of quoting statistics.

It's true that cancers usually grow relatively slowly, but logic dictates that at some point they will spread, and the longer the delay, the greater likelihood of this.

So what could I do? I had to start taking control.

I took a deep breath. Until now I'd been unable to focus on learning about my cancer and the potential treatments as I was still in denial and shock. But now I had to; I had to study the various surgical options, their benefits and the drawbacks both on my chances of cure and on my final appearance. Then I had to work out how to get my best option. The delayed operation date meant that I had little to lose by exploring other possibilities, including surgeons and operations. There was little to lose, and much to be gained.

So I spent the next forty-eight hours on the Internet, looking mainly at cancer charity websites and patient's forums. I spoke to my friend's two kids, who were

both doctors—one in plastic surgery, the other a radiologist in a well-known cancer hospital. They provided useful advice and support, and so did the internet. Two days later, on the Friday, I was confident of my best options. I definitely wanted a 'DIEP flap operation' (boob job with tummy tuck).

A national newspaper had run an article, ranking surgeons who could do this specialised procedure, based on the views of their peers. It was available on the internet, and these seemed as good credentials as any, so I chose a surgeon, Mr Page, who scored well and who worked within commutable distance of my home.

Armed with a plan, I emailed Nurse Eileen. I asked to be referred to Mr Page, for a DIEP flap.

Half an hour later, she phoned,

'Hello dear, I think you have made a good choice. Mr Page is excellent. I've had a word with Miss Gomez. She says you need to get your GP to do the referral.'

'OK Eileen, thanks so much for getting back to me so quickly.' That woman was amazing. I knew she'd have been really busy as usual. But she clearly understood that I would be in agonies all weekend if I didn't hear back. She didn't make me feel embarrassed that I'd decided to go somewhere else for my surgery either.

I said goodbye to Eileen and managed to get an appointment with my GP that afternoon. I was on a roll.

'Hello, what can I do for you?' as before, my GP was staring absentmindedly at his computer.

Hadn't he read my notes?

'I think you'd better read the letter from the hospital.'

He turned to me sharply with a surprised look. I saw his expression change again, as he read. I guessed he'd reached the bit about me having breast cancer.

'Oh. I see. How are you?'

I briefly explained about the weeks of tests, the delayed operation, and that Miss Gomez could not offer me the operation I wanted. I asked him if he would refer me to Mr Page.

'I sympathise, but Miss Gomez will need to refer you.'

'But she told me I had to ask you.' I was losing patience, and I was in no mood for playing 'pass the patient.' As far as I was concerned, the music had stopped with him, and he needed to help me.

'Well of course I can refer you, but I don't have any of your results. It would've been much better for Miss Gomez to communicate with the new surgeon directly.'

'Perhaps, but she won't.'

'Well, I think that's ridiculous, but don't worry, I'll arrange the referral for you.'

'Can I just check? Will you write to Mr Page directly?' I asked. 'I don't want to get stuck in the 'Choose and Book' system and lose time.'

I knew from past experience that my GP used the NHS Choose and Book system for referring patients. I'd encountered problems with it before. It seemed to just offer appointments for hospitals within the region, and I didn't want to wait two more precious weeks only to receive a computerized invitation to contact my original hospital for an appointment. I was in a more assertive state than I'd been since I'd received my diagnosis, and I wasn't in the mood for any administrative delays.

'OK, I'll write directly to the surgeon. It'll cost the practice more because we're penalized for referrals outside our area, but don't worry, I'm not an accountant and we need to do what's best for you.'

'Good. Thanks.'

I handed him a sheet of paper on which I'd copied Mr Page's name and the hospital address (courtesy of Google), and left.

I unlocked the front door and walked into the kitchen.

Another Friday evening, another weekend of anxious limbo. I opened a bottle of red, sat on the sofa and messaged my daughter. We had a long discussion about the NHS. She was as shocked as me that I'd been put in this position. Then I phoned my son and updated him, then I called Phil and a few other close friends who were anxiously following my progress. I turned on the TV, but I couldn't really concentrate.

The next morning I woke early. I couldn't settle. I got dressed and jogged to the park. I tried to distract myself with some hill runs, but my mind was racing far faster than my legs.

My son and daughter-in-law had invited me for a barbecue. It was just what I needed—a few hours to forget my anxious limbo.

By Sunday I needed to do something ... anything. I must've been asleep behind a bush when God handed out patience, and I'm never any good at waiting. I surfed the net and, remarkably, found Mr Page's personal email address. I wrestled with myself—I couldn't contact him directly, could I? How could I be that cheeky? I should wait until Monday and speak to his secretary, not the Great Man himself?

But in the end desperation won over perceived protocol and I sent him an email explaining my predicament and the delay, and asking him how I could best expedite an appointment with him.

I didn't know whether he'd read my email or reply to it, but at least I'd done everything I could before Monday morning when the working world would spring into action again.

Monday morning I was up early. I glanced through my emails. There was one from Mr Page, sent at 7am. I caught my breath, then opened it:

'Thank you for your message Dr Thompson.

I'm sorry to hear about your cancer.

Your GP will need to refer you to one of the breast surgeons first, and they will refer you to me if appropriate.

I have copied my PA and the lead breast care nurse into this email so that they can assist you in expediting this referral.

Best wishes,

Mark Page'

I was touched that he'd replied personally and promptly, but sadly neither the lead breast care nurse nor his PA ever contacted me as he'd requested.

However, his succinct email provided key information. I needed to get my GP to change the referral to one of the breast surgeons who worked with Mr Page.

I searched the internet again for the names of the breast surgeons at his hospital. There were two—Mr Parsons and Mrs Grant. I phoned the hospital and spoke to someone in the consultants' office.

'Oh yes, Mr Parsons is away on holiday, but Mrs Grant doesn't have a waiting list. If your GP could fax the letter to this number we can sort the appointment.'

Great, things were starting to look good. No waiting list. Hardly believing my luck, I phoned my GP's secretary.

'Oh, he hasn't written the referral letter yet, but as soon as he does I'll fax it to Mrs Grant's secretary, and I'll phone you to let you know it's gone.'

I took a deep breath and suppressed my frustration that the letter hadn't been written yet. 'Would it help if I dropped in a summary of what has happened to me, to help him write the letter?' I asked.

'Oh yes, I'm sure it would. Can you drop it into reception?'

I typed up a summary of everything that had happened and ran with it to the surgery. I was effectively writing my own referral letter, having already researched which consultant I needed. Surely I was doing my GP's job? Whatever, at least if

I did it, it would be done right.

I waited and waited. Eventually, around 2pm his secretary phoned to say the letter had been faxed.

Thanking her, I put the phone down and immediately phoned Mrs Grant's secretary.

'Hello, I think you've just received a fax from my GP. I was hoping to make an appointment with Mrs Grant.'

'Oh, yes, I can give you an appointment on 8th June.'

I lead ball dropped into the pit of my stomach again. 'But that's not for two and a half weeks. Your colleague this morning said there wasn't any waiting list? I need to explain; I have to be seen sooner than that. There were delays at the first hospital I went to and now it's over ten weeks since I discovered the cancer. I can't wait another two and a half weeks before I even see her.'

'I'm afraid I can't do anything to help. With the bank holidays coming up we lose two clinics. This week's clinic already has too many patients, and I'm not allowed to add extras.'

'You said the clinic was overbooked, so that means you must squeeze some extras in. Can't you fit me in somehow?'

'No, I've told you, I'm not allowed to overbook.' She sounded irritated, I could tell that smart-arse arguments wouldn't work. I tried a different tack,

'Well what about private appointments?'

I only needed to see Mrs Grant so that she could refer me to Mr Page, so if I paid for one private appointment I could save time. I could find the money for that, it was so important.

'The first private appointment is two days after the first NHS appointment.' Her voice softened, 'Look, I really can't fit you in any sooner. I would strongly advise you to take the NHS appointment, because it's the first one available, and there's only the one appointment left for that clinic. If you don't grab it, it'll be gone.'

'OK, thanks. I'll take it, but if there are any cancellations could you let me know?"

'Yes, I will, but it's really unlikely. People hardly ever cancel for this clinic.'

I put the phone down. The 8th of June was two and a half weeks away. Not great, but what could I do?

So that's how I decided on what operation was best, who was the best surgeon, and how I arranged an NHS appointment at the right hospital. Looking back, my GP was correct. Miss Gomez could—and should—have referred me directly to Mr Page or a plastic surgeon with similar expertise. This would have avoided my having to start again with another breast surgeon in order to be referred to Mr Page. However, as it turned out, it was probably for the best that I saw Mrs. Grant.

As you'll have noticed, my preferred style was non-confrontational, and to rely on the doctor to decide on my treatment. It was only when forced to that I took control. In similar circumstances some people react differently. Some absolutely need to be in control of all medical decisions. For this reason, different consultants suit different people. Neither approach is right or wrong, and your needs may change along the course of your treatment. However, from my observations, I would say that the people who take control generally get better care. They're not afraid to make demands and challenge decisions. They're harder to deal with, but people who demand usually get what they want, as I was to discover later.

Summary:

Modern breast cancer treatment in the UK and most developed countries aims not only to treat the cancer most effectively, but to minimise cosmetic damage Everyone in the UK has a right to be offered the best treatment for their cancer in a timely fashion. If that treatment is not available locally, you should be given the opportunity to receive the treatment elsewhere.

If you are not happy with the treatment offered, don't just accept it. There are various ways to challenge medical decisions, including having a second opinion, and, if all else fails, there is an official complaint procedure.

Generally people respond positively if you voice your unhappiness. The worst thing you can do is smile and say nothing. Both the quality and quantity of your life may suffer if you don't speak out.

You may not feel like reading about your cancer. That is normal, but as soon as you feel strong enough, you should learn as much as you can about your cancer type and the possible treatments. In the end, you have the most interest in ensuring you get the best care, and knowledge really is power.

Further Information:

NICE Guidelines CG80   http://goo.gl/JGzAwB
NICE Guidelines CG81   http://goo.gl/8SK6Ee
What is PALS? (NHS)   http://bit.ly/1OjPnAK

Making a Complaint (NHS)   http://bit.ly/18zciXt

Chapter 15

Second opinions

So, in the end, I didn't accept the incomplete options I'd been offered. In my case the delayed operation forced me to look at alternatives. Nobody had suggested that I request a second opinion, nobody told me I could choose a surgeon outside my health region, but all these options were there.

What is a second opinion? It means being seen by a different specialist, who will make an independent assessment of your medical situation and what treatment would be best for you. Their opinion may confirm the opinion of the first doctor, or may conflict with it.

Legally you don't have an automatic right to a second opinion, but most GPs will not refuse to arrange it without good reason, and people are sent for second opinions fairly regularly.

So, if you have concerns about treatment you've received from a consultant, you can ask your GP to arrange for you have a second opinion.

But it isn't easy, is it? Requesting a second opinion has negative connotations in British culture. The implication is that you're questioning your doctor's decisions—even insulting them. It's almost on a par with changing your hairdresser.

You don't know what I mean? Yes you do. Have you ever actually changed your hairdresser? Even when they've continued to plough on with the same unflattering style for you every time you go, regardless of their reassurances to the contrary? And if you have eventually taken that drastic step, did you just tell your hairdresser you were changing, or did you feel compelled to make an excuse, such as you were moving to Azerbaijan, or you were due to have a large operation which would preclude any haircuts for at least a year, or you'd developed a life-threatening allergy to hair spray and had been forbidden to step within 100 yards of any hairdressing salon?

Sound at all familiar? At least a bad hair-do will eventually grow out.

The North American culture is quite different. People have more control over which doctor or specialist they see, and are often well-informed about their options, and have firm opinions as to what they want. Generally they have no embarrassment at changing doctors (They probably don't worry about changing their hairdressers either).

I want to reassure you that it is perfectly acceptable to ask for a second opinion if you ever have any doubts about your medical care. Of course the down side is that referring you to a new consultant takes time, which may be an important factor if you have cancer. Even so, changing horses (as I fondly think of my brothers in the medical profession) mid-course may still be your best option, so don't dismiss the idea.

My Story

I spent the next two weeks worrying. I'd booked a week's holiday at the end of May. In the end I didn't go, and forfeited the money—what if a cancellation for the clinic came up whilst I was away? It just wasn't worth the risk.

I wanted to make sure that the new consultant had all my test reports; the mammogram, the pathology reports and the MRI scans. I didn't want any more obstacles getting in the way of my operation. I telephoned Miss Gomez's secretary and left her a message, asking her if she could send the information to Mrs Grant.

The week before my appointment, I hadn't heard back. I phoned the Breast Care nurses' number and asked for Eileen.

'Sorry, Eileen isn't available – can I help? This is Cheryl, Breast Care Nurse Practitioner, speaking.'

'Hello Cheryl, I'm seeing Mrs Grant next week. I left a message with Miss Gomez' secretary about getting my test results and scans to her. I haven't heard anything so I just wanted to make sure she'd sent them?'

'She's been on holiday so she probably hasn't seen your message.' Cheryl's voice was flat, unhelpful.

'Well I do need the results to be transferred. I can come and collect the scans if it makes it easier?'

'That's probably not possible. We'd have to make a special request for the MRI

scan. I'm afraid it'll all take a while.'

'But my appointment's next week.'

'Sorry, there's nothing I can do.'

'Look, I need the results. Surely there's some way around this? Is Eileen available?'

'I don't think so. I'll let Eileen know you called – she's busy right now. Bye.'

I was shaking with frustration, anger and impotence. Did she have any idea what she was doing to me? How important this was? This was my survival that she couldn't be bothered to help with.

Just as the pent-up emotions and stress expanded and exploded through my body, my phone rang,

'Hello dear, this is Eileen. I've just heard you need your scans and pathology reports. Don't worry, I'm on the case. I'll phone you back when it's sorted.'

I was still shaking, but gently now—thank God for Eileen. Half an hour later she phoned again. 'Right dear, I've arranged for the MRI scan to be emailed to Mrs Grant, together with the pathology reports. The mammogram isn't digital though, so I'm getting a copy. Could you pop in and collect it? I know it's a bit of a way for you to come?'

'Yes Eileen, of course. I'll come first thing tomorrow, thanks so much.'

'Absolutely no problem, dear. It's important Mrs Grant has all this information. Bye now, and good luck with your appointment.'

By now I was in a permanent state of anxiety. I tried to keep as fit as possible, partly to distract myself, but also to keep myself in good shape for the operation. I had lots of non-productive days too though. My mind was bouncing around like a kid on a space-hopper.

Then, half-way through the wait, as I was wheeling my supermarket trolley firmly past the biscuit aisle, my mobile rang.

'Hello, is that Mrs Thompson? This is Brenda from the Breast Care unit. Miss Gomez has asked me to phone you. An earlier operation slot has become available in mid-June, would you like it?'

My mind lurched clumsily from special offers to specialist care.

'Wow. That's a surprise. I never expected that.'

I was in a quandary. Should I grab the earlier date for my life-saving surgery, with the less-than-ideal operation, or should I continue to wait for the appointment with the new consultant, not knowing what the outcome would be?

I felt I was playing some strange game of snakes and ladders—where the stakes were my life. My brain was paralysed with indecision.

In the end I decided to be honest, and I explained my dilemma. Brenda made a suggestion, which I would never have dared to consider—that I accept the earlier operation date, but in the meantime still go ahead with my visit to the new consultant.

It's strange, my life and body were on the line, and yet I still felt I should play fair. I didn't feel entitled to keep both options open. I desperately needed to become more demanding and assertive, but it was so hard. I should have found it easier than most—I was a doctor after all, this was my playing field. But even I didn't know the rules of this new game, and I was so nervous of throwing the wrong number, sliding down a snake and losing everything.

So now I had an earlier operation slot AND a chance to see a new consultant as well as the chance of a more suitable operation for my needs. Things were looking up.

I realised my fingers were gripping my supermarket trolley, which was blocking an elderly woman from reaching the Rich Teas, 'Oh sorry.'

I moved the trolley. Right, back to fruit and veg section. What did I need? Oh yes, onions and an aubergine. And maybe a toffee praline ice-cream. Well it was on special offer.

I spent the weekend before my appointment with Mrs Grant studying. My whole future depended on this new consultant accepting me as a patient. Somehow I had to convince her that I was worth it (or so I felt).

All sorts of fears popped into my mind. What if she told me I was too old for the DIEP operation? That it wasn't intended for middle-aged past-their-sell-by-date cookies like me. What if she told me that she had a long list of seriously-ill women wanting operations, and I should go back to Miss Gomez? What if, what if, what if?

I practiced what I would say to her again and again. Most surgeons I knew had short attention spans. If you didn't get your message across in the first 30 seconds, their eyes would just glaze over. I needed a succinct and compelling reason why she should take over my care. I had to 'sell' my case. I had to distil a complex, convoluted series of events into a simple summary. I studied the copies of all the letters from the hospital to my GP. I made notes. I rehearsed, again and again.

At last the day of the appointment arrived. Phil came with me. We set off with lots of time. We had a coffee at the station. The train arrived and we found two empty seats.

We sat on the stationary train and waited, and waited. Finally, fifteen minutes late, the public address system crackled:

'I'm sorry, we have no idea where the driver has gone. Your best bet is to just get the next train out of here and change at another station. We do apologise for any inconvenience.'

'What the…?' Phil's face was turning a strange colour and he was visibly shaking.

'Come on, there's nothing we can do. Let's find another train.'

After a sharp exchange of words between Phil and the ticket collector, we got on the suggested train, which would take us vaguely in the right direction. After changing trains again we eventually got off at a station a good mile from the hospital, with very little time and no further transport options apart from our legs. This wasn't quite how I'd envisaged putting the benefits of getting myself fit for my operation to good use.

With minutes to spare we arrived at the hospital and found the outpatients clinic. Feeling very sweaty from my unscheduled sprint, I freshened up in the ladies as best I could.

I joined Phil back in the waiting room, but didn't bother with the magazines. I was too busy rehearsing the summary of the case for the defense. Phil understood, and for once he didn't feel obliged to rack his brain for jokes to keep me smiling.

After twenty minutes a nurse called me into a consultation room. A petite, oriental lady, perhaps in her early forties greeted me, 'Hello, I am Mrs Grant. Please do sit down.' She had a real presence, an aura—or maybe that was just my perception, because to me she was God. She could make or break my future, or lack of one, in the next ten minutes.

I felt like a medical student preparing to present a patient's case history to my consultant – which was exactly what I was doing, come to think of it, only this time the patient was me. I grasped my notes as if they were the secret of life—I didn't dare speak without them for fear of forgetting some critical fact, losing my case and being cast out of this Centre of Excellence, deprived of all the opportunities for optimal treatment which it represented.

Mrs Grant smiled, 'I see you're a doctor. Are you a medical doctor?'

'Yes. I was a paediatrician, but now I work in research, in the pharmaceutical industry.'

'Really? What company do you work for? What drugs have you worked on?'
She seemed oblivious of the enormity of the situation. Her relaxed, interested
manner threw me, she wasn't the archetypal surgeon I was expecting. I was so
focused on making my case that my mind went blank at her chatty questions. I
couldn't remember one drug I'd worked on over the past twenty years. I even had
difficulty remembering any of the companies I'd worked for. I started to worry
that she'd think I was a half-wit, as I struggled to make any intelligent response.

Eventually I said, 'I know you're busy so I won't waste your time with small
talk.'

'Oh I've lots of time today. The clinic's usually much busier than this.' she
smiled again. 'So tell me why you want a second opinion?'

I related what had happened to me, reading from my notes throughout.
Eventually I finished off:

'I don't actually want a second opinion. I do feel that Miss Gomez did a
competent and careful assessment of my cancer. The reason I'm here is because
her unit is two surgeons down, so there's a two month delay before my operation,
and in addition, she can't offer me the DIEP operation that I would really like.'

I held my breath as I waited for her response.

Mrs Grant had been listening intently, leaning forward in her seat, interrupting
with questions occasionally as I spoke.

'I see. Right, would you mind if I examine you, Dr Thompson?'

'No, of course not.' I almost shouted, jumping out of my chair as if it had
delivered 240 volts to my bottom, and ripping my jumper and bra off.

'That's fine, plenty of time.' she grinned.

Afterwards, she waited for me to get dressed, and once I was sitting back next
to Phil, she started to talk.

'A mastectomy with an implant would be completely the wrong operation for
you. Implants are more suitable for younger women, they just don't look natural
on women of your age, and it wouldn't match your other breast.' She paused,
then continued:

'I'm confident that I can remove your tumour with a Wide Local Excision, and
I would reduce the size of your other breast in the same operation so that you'd
be symmetrical. Alternatively, if you prefer, I can perform a mastectomy. In this
case I would discuss your case with Mr Page, and ask him to perform a DIEP
reconstruction at the same time.'

She started to explain the DIEP operation, but I interrupted.

'It's OK, I understand what's involved.'

'Ah yes, of course I was forgetting you're a doctor.'

'Can I ask about the wide local excision? How do you know that my right breast won't shrink to be smaller than my left after radiotherapy?' I was thinking of Miss Gomez's rationale for delaying the operation to make my normal breast smaller.

'I don't, but I'd make your left breast slightly smaller than your right to allow for that. It's difficult to predict how much your breast will shrink, but if the worst came to the worst we could always operate on your left breast again to adjust the size.'

I felt so comfortable with this woman. She was so calm. She acted as if she had all day to talk to me. She encouraged me to tell her everything. She respected my professional position without appearing threatened. What's more, I felt totally confident that she would do the best operation for me.

She had started off confirming my fear that the implant was the wrong operation for me.

She had portrayed the Wide Local Excision in a much more positive light than Miss Gomez and, importantly, she was prepared to operate on my normal breast at the same time, so I wouldn't be left lopsided until some indeterminate time after my radiotherapy. In view of the long delay before Miss Gomez could even offer me a cancer operation, it seemed doubtful that a purely cosmetic operation on my normal breast would have had much priority. The idea of waking up looking normal and ready to start my new post-cancer life was important.

I desperately wanted Mrs Grant to be my surgeon.

She paused. 'So, did you just want a second opinion, or did you want me to take over your care?' She was very professional, asking the second part of the question very quietly, casually. I sensed that she would never 'poach' a patient from a colleague. However the question seemed ludicrous to me. I would have killed to be under her care. I tried to sound casual too, as I replied.

'I would like you to take over my care.'

'I won't be able to perform the operation any sooner than you would have had it under Miss Gomez, but I don't know why you're so anxious about the time. You don't need to worry.' she said in her calm, even voice.

It's true, I was anxious about the timescale, but the type of operation available to me was also important, and I felt much more confident with what she was offering. If she found at the operation that she couldn't remove all the tumour,

I could be seen immediately by Mr Page, in the same hospital, and have a mastectomy with DIEP reconstruction as a follow-on procedure. Either of these options would give good cosmetic results and would leave me looking 'normal' right away.

She turned to the computer on her desk,

'Let's get you booked in then, so you have a slot reserved.'

She turned to the nurse. 'Can you take Dr Thompson to see Monica?'

Then, turning back to me, 'Monica's one of our Breast Care Nurses. She'll have a chat with you.'

'Thank you so much, Mrs Grant. Thank you so much for taking me on. I feel so much happier now.'

She grinned and waved me out of the door, just in time to stop me collapsing at her feet and hugging her legs.

I followed the nurse into another room, where a dark-haired woman in her early thirties was sitting at a computer.

'Hello, come and sit down. I'm Monica. I'm a Breast Care Nurse Practitioner.'

She talked to me for about 10 minutes. She was pleasant. She wasn't Eileen, but then Eileen was a very hard act to follow. Still, what did it matter? I had Mrs Grant as my surgeon. I was blessed.

So, I'd refused the wide local excision (WLE) operation when Miss Gomez offered it, but ended up accepting it happily from Mrs Grant. A woman's prerogative to change her mind? Yes and no. There are many factors which affect decision-making when you have a serious illness.

Firstly the two consultants presented the operation very differently—or at least that was my perception. In the words of the French novelist Gustave Flaubert (no, I hadn't heard of him either) 'There is no truth. There is only perception.'

My perception from Miss Gomez was that the WLE would leave scarring inside my breast, which would form lumps at future dates, and these would therefore need to be checked for cancer, plus my breast would become shrunken with the radiotherapy. Mrs Grant had commented that it was always preferable to keep your own breast tissue, and therefore WLE was a good option, and she had offered to make the other breast the same size during the same operation.

Both surgeons had given me correct information. Miss Gomez had, quite reasonably, taken pains to warn me of the long-term effects, which had made the outcome sound worse than when Mrs Grant described it.

Our decisions can be influenced by our own perceptions of what we hear, and by the way someone presents the information (which is why companies have large marketing departments).

If, when Mrs Grant did the operation, she found that she wasn't able to remove the tumour completely, I would be able to have my choice of mastectomy and reconstruction, through her links with Mr Page.

Regarding the delay in surgery, Miss Gomez seemed to share my concern that the wait was too long, but she was powerless to shorten it. Mrs Grant seemed more relaxed about the delay. Either way, even with the weeks lost while I had waited for the second opinion, my new operation date was not delayed beyond the original date Miss Gomez had been able to offer.

Summary:

It is reasonable to request a second opinion from a different consultant within the NHS if you have concerns about the treatment or advice you have been offered. If you wish to switch doctors, or just get a second opinion, do ask. Generally people will not think badly of you, and even if they do, their opinion is not as important as your well-being.

Unlike some other cultures, British people are very reluctant to question their medical treatment and ask to see another doctor.

People who unashamedly demand the best for themselves, and who are not frightened of appearing belligerent or being unpopular, usually get what they want. A doctor may be very competent, but you need to have confidence in them.

Whilst being prepared to challenge any medical advice/treatment offered is important, equally don't forget that your doctor may understand the situation better than you do, and at least consider their advice carefully.

A second opinion will usually introduce a delay—but sometimes it is still worth it.

Further Information:

The NHS Constitution	http://bit.ly/1kQMX03
Second Opinions (NHS)	http://bit.ly/1Qzj443
Citizens Advice	http://goo.gl/XQ0TtI

Chapter 16

The operation and informed consent

Most people with breast cancer will end up having some type of surgery. The surgery will depend on the situation, but will often involve either removal of the lump, removal of the whole breast (mastectomy), or sometimes both breasts. In addition, either a sentinel lymph node biopsy will be taken, or your surgeon may decide to remove more lymph nodes from around your breast, such as the armpit, if the cancer has already spread to them.

If too many lymph nodes are removed from your armpit, there's a risk of lymphoedema, a permanent swelling of the arm, so it is important to find out whether it is necessary. A sentinel lymph node biopsy is a clever technique to determine whether the cancer has spread to the lymphatic system. By injecting radioactive material, (and sometimes blue dye), into the affected breast, the radioactivity (or dye) will spread to the lymph nodes in the same way that a cancer will spread.

The first lymph node the cancer (or radioactivity and dye) would reach is called the sentinel node, and this can be detected with a radiation detector and then removed at operation. If the sentinel node is found to be clear of cancer, it can be assumed that the other lymph nodes are all clear too. However, if cancer is found in the sentinel node, then more lymph nodes will need to be removed and tested.

If you have a wide local excision (removal of the cancer lump only) with a sentinel node biopsy, you will have quite a busy time on operation day. Not only do you need to have the radioactivity injection to locate the sentinel lymph node, but you may need to have small wires put into your breast, using X-ray guidance, so that the surgeon knows exactly where the cancer is when they operate. (Exactly where the cancer finishes and normal breast tissue starts isn't always easy to see during the operation, and it is important not to leave any cancer behind).

The procedure for mastectomy will be different and depends on your particular cancer. You may choose to have an immediate reconstruction, and, provided there is no medical reason why you can't have this, you will wake up with two normal breasts. If you don't have this, you will wake up with a flat area where your breast was. More information sources on this can be found at the end of the chapter.

Before any operation, or any other important procedure, your doctor needs to explain to you what exactly will be done, and what the possible side-effects may be, even the rare and unlikely ones. They should give you a written summary of what they have told you and allow you time to read it, consider it and discuss it with anyone you wish before you sign it. This is called giving Informed Consent, and the consent form is an important legal document.

I experienced many different variations of the consent signing procedure during my cancer treatment. Mrs Grant explained what she would do when she first saw me. Then she brought me back a couple of weeks afterwards, when one of her registrars went through the consent form in detail and gave me time to ask questions. Finally I signed the form and received a copy for myself. This is an excellent example of how informed consent should be taken. If you're not given an adequate explanation, or offered enough time to ask questions, or if you're not encouraged to read the consent form through before signing, you should politely request this. It is your right, and a very important one. You are making a decision about your life, not whether to accept terms and conditions for the latest iTunes update.

My Story

The day after seeing Mrs Grant, I phoned Eileen and explained that I wouldn't need the operation slot with Miss Gomez. I knew how precious those slots were from my own anguish.

Eileen was supportive as always, 'Mrs Grant's an excellent surgeon. You'll be fine there. Yes, I know you wanted the option of the DIEP operation, so you need to go there. You'll be in good hands. Thanks so much for letting us know. Please do let me know how things go, Kathleen.'

She never made me feel awkward or disloyal for jumping ships. I was very grateful for her mature understanding.

I spent the next four weeks counting the days. I just wanted to get the operation over with.

I did lots of exercise. I was determined to look fitter and healthier than every other patient in the hospital when I went for my operation. I wanted to be toned and sun-tanned. I wanted people to look at me and think I was in the wrong hospital, that I couldn't possibly have cancer. It was my way of fighting, and one of the few things still within my control.

A friend gave me Reiki healing sessions. I would lie on her couch for an hour, drifting off into a semi-conscious state. I always left her studio feeling stronger and refreshed.

During that time Phil moved away to the South coast. I helped him pack. He told me he would come and stay with me for my operation though. 'Keep smiling,' he winked, and drove off. Our lives had moved on from what had once been, he was now a good friend and I appreciated his support.

A couple of weeks into this waiting period, I received a letter, apparently from my GP's surgery, inviting me for a routine screening mammogram. I was surprised at how upsetting I found this. My GP knew that I was waiting for an operation for breast cancer. I couldn't understand why they had sent it. It took me two days to steel myself just to phone the telephone number on the letter and explain why I wouldn't be attending.

I phoned during the stated office hours, but there was no reply, and no voice mail. Feeling upset and frustrated, I wrote a letter instead, and posted it through the surgery letter-box, as this was the address given on the letter.

A week or so later I received a letter from the Head of the Breast Screening Unit, chastising me for not attending the mammogram and not letting them know.

I replied, explaining that I had let them know, and I suggested that they liaise with GPs to ensure that letters weren't sent out inappropriately to women newly diagnosed with breast cancer.

I later received a reply from the Programme Director, apologizing. The letter included a form for me to sign, to opt out of the screening programme, stating that if I signed the form, I wouldn't get any further distressing mammogram invitations. It failed to mention that, five years after my operation, I would need to revert back to this screening programme, for future cancer surveillance. If I'd signed this waiver, I would have been excluded from this. I was and am shocked that I was encouraged to do this without an explanation of the consequences.

At last the day before my operation arrived. Phil had come up to stay, as promised. That night, we went to an Italian restaurant for dinner.

'Any wine?' he asked.

'I shouldn't really, before the operation, should I?'

'Well let's not order a bottle, but I'm sure a glass won't hurt.'

I relaxed over the pasta and deep red Barolo. It was hard to believe that I was going to have major surgery the following day.

In fact I relaxed so much that Phil had to be quite firm about me not ordering a second glass,

'No, Kathleen. Hangovers and operations don't mix. You'll regret it if you do.'

I slept surprisingly well that night.

The next morning I got up early and had a light breakfast before 7am as instructed.

We reported to the Pre-operative Unit at 8.30am. The operation was scheduled for early afternoon, but before that I needed my radio-isotope scan to locate my sentinel lymph nodes, and after that I was to go to the radiology department, so the radiologist could insert wires into my breast, to show Mrs Grant exactly where the tumour started and finished.

PATIENTS THIS SIDE

This strange sign greeted us as we entered the Radio-isotope Department.

'Oh, can't we sit together?' Phil asked, looking puzzled.

'Yes I think we can. The sign's probably intended to separate the patients who've been injected with radio-active material, to protect everyone else from too much radioactivity. I haven't been injected yet.'

I reported at the reception desk and then I made a tea for Phil from the small tray provided. I was still allowed clear fluids, but I wasn't really thirsty. We sat and waited.

'Kathleen Thompson?'

'Yes'

The technician led me into a room with what looked like an X-ray machine in the middle, but it was actually a huge Geiger counter, for detecting radioactivity.

'*Could you pop this blue gown on please – opening down the front?*
I did as I was told.
'*That's great. Now can I get you to lie on this couch?*
'*OK. I'm going to inject some radioactive liquid into your breast. It is your right breast, isn't it?*'
'*Yes it is.*' *She brandished a small syringe of clear liquid,*
'*Right, well, when I inject this, it'll travel along lymph channels to your lymph nodes. The nodes it reaches first are what we call the sentinel lymph nodes. Usually they're in your armpit, but every now and then they're somewhere else, like above your collar bone.*

'*Anyway, this big machine you're lying under will find that first node by detecting the radioactivity. I'll mark the spot where the radioactivity is the strongest, and your sentinel lymph nodes should be directly under that mark. Do you understand?*'
'*Yes thanks.*'
'*OK, well here comes the injection. It'll be a bit sore, but try to lie still if you can.*'

She stuck the needle into me, near my nipple, and started injecting the innocuous-looking clear liquid into my breast. Then she moved my arm so that it was lying above my head, to expose my armpit to the machine, and asked me to stay very still, before disappearing behind a screen.

The machine started to move slowly above me. As I lay there, I had nothing to do but think. I thought how lucky I was to have access to all these expensive machines. The mammography machine, MRI scanners, and now this radiation scanner. They were all worth hundreds of thousands of pounds. If I'd been born in a third world country, my story would have been very different—and much shorter.

I must admit, after thinking these deep philosophical muses, I was slightly underwhelmed when the culmination of this sophisticated procedure involved the technician drawing a large cross just below my armpit with a biro.

Having been duly marked up, I went back to the pre-op unit. My next appointment was the radiology department, for the wires insertion.

The tall nurse behind the desk smiled,
'*Oh hello, you're back. The X-ray department's just called. Your appointment's delayed until 11 o'clock. But don't worry – everything's fine.*'

Why did she say '*But everything's fine?*' There was something about the way she said it... I subconsciously clocked it.

'By the way, they're hoping to start your operation a little early; maybe 1.30pm. In the meantime just make yourself comfortable in the waiting room until we have a bed ready for you. Remember, nothing to eat or drink though.'

Phil and I sat and chatted, but after a while I suggested he went. There was little he could do now. I just had to wait for the X-ray and then the surgery, and he wouldn't be able to come with me for either of those procedures. The waiting was all a bit of an anti-climax after the rush, and to be honest we were both running out of conversation and energy.

'OK, I'll get off then. Now are you sure you don't want me to visit tonight? I can always cancel my other plans.'

'No, it's fine. Mickie and Joe are coming so I'll have plenty of company.'

'OK then, well, chin up.'

After he'd gone I texted my son and daughter:

'Hi both, Good news! They're starting my operation early, so I expect I'll be back on the ward by about 4pm. I should be awake when you come to visit tonight. Mum xxx'

Thirty minutes later another nurse came to tell me my X-ray procedure would be delayed until 1pm. 'But don't worry, it isn't a problem, and you can go straight from X-ray to theatre.'

I suppose my suspicions should have been alerted by the constant reassurances that there wasn't a problem. I was getting pretty bored by then. There wasn't much to do in the little waiting room, and the tray of coffee and biscuits was out of bounds. There were still no beds free for me, and they didn't seem in a hurry to get me ready for theatre.

Around 12 o'clock a wave of panic ran through the nurses. They whisked me into the ward, a bed having miraculously become available, and pulled a curtain around me. 'The surgical team are here to mark you up for your operation.' The bubbly dark-haired nurse informed me in a hallowed whisper.

I hurriedly stripped to the waist. I was getting into the habit of baring my chest to every new stranger I met. In fact, I was slightly concerned that I might absent-mindedly start doing this out there in the real world. I climbed onto the bed and waited for the surgical team.

Then I heard Mrs. Grant's voice on the other side of the curtain. It sounded as if she was on the phone.

Because hospital curtains block the view of the person behind them, people sometimes forget that there's someone there, but those curtains are certainly not sound-proof.

'I'm not starting a four hour operation at 3pm. That's ridiculous.' She was talking quietly but I could hear the anger in her voice.

I was puzzled. Was someone asking her to do another operation after mine? Something wasn't right... I forced my hands to relax —they seemed to be gripping the sheet very tightly.

She finished her call, then she phoned someone else. It sounded like her secretary. 'Hello Audrey, could you put me through to Dr. Frimley please?' (I knew he was one of the radiologists.)

'David, it's Victoria. You've heard about the problem with localizing one of my patients?'

Did she mean that my X-ray procedure had been delayed because they hadn't been able to locate me? I know I was a bit late back from the radio-isotope department, but the nurse had said it was fine, and I'd been waiting here ever since?

Then, as I listened more, things started to make sense. The 'localization' she was talking about was the name of the X-ray procedure I was waiting for. So she WAS talking about me, and there WAS a problem. My chest and throat felt tight. Suddenly I felt cold and clammy, despite the heat of the ward. Surely there wasn't a hitch at this late stage? Not after all I'd been through to get this operation?

Her voice faded, she must have moved away, and, although straining to listen, I couldn't hear any more. I sat there semi-naked, shivering and terrified.

Then the curtains moved apart and a tall man with short blond hair and fine features appeared in the gap. He was dressed in theatre 'greens'.

'Hello. I'm Michael Swann, Mrs Grant's registrar.' He paused. 'I'm supposed to mark you up for surgery, but I expect you've heard about this X-ray problem?'

I made a non-committal reply. I wanted to find out what was happening and I didn't want to discourage him from spilling as many beans as I could coax from him.

He carried on: 'Well, as there aren't any radiologists free to do your localization, we'll probably just remove your sentinel lymph nodes today. We can reschedule the tumour removal for another day.' His voice was casual, as if he was telling me that they'd run out of cheese burgers, so I'd have to make do with a sausage roll.

The brightness of the ward seemed to dim as he spoke. I could no longer hear the nurses bustling. I seemed to be falling backwards into a silent darkness. My *life-saving operation, which I'd been focusing on for all those long weeks, was now fading and shrinking, disappearing before my eyes like a mirage once again.*

I remember attending an assertiveness course once: the tutor described a scenario where various people did annoying things to a victim throughout the day—spilled coffee on his computer, helped themselves to his pens, scratched his desk, forgot to invite him to an important meeting, and every time they said 'Oh, sorry', and he just smiled and said 'that's OK, not a problem'. By the end of the day he was so wound up by all these events that when he came home and his small son wiped ice-cream on his suit he just exploded in anger. All his pent-up annoyances from all the other events were vented on his son.

Well this unfortunate registrar became the recipient of all my frustration of weeks and weeks of delays and obstacles.

'Are you telling me you're not going to remove my tumour today? I've been waiting over three months for this operation. I've a large tumour which needs removing. Someone's travelled a hundred miles to stay with me and he's arranged everything in his diary around this operation date. You're telling me you're going to subject me to two operations, and two anaesthetics—with all the associated risks—when one would have done? Don't you realize I've been focused on this day for weeks? My whole life has revolved around it. Have you any idea how devastated I'm feeling right now?'

My voice was getting louder and louder. My eyes filled with tears of frustration and fear. I couldn't believe I'd gone through so much to get to this moment, and now they were going to take it all away from me. Just when the finishing line was in sight, I was going to be flung back into limbo. And how long would it be before they could fit me in for the rescheduled operation? Another four weeks? But of course 'delay doesn't matter'. Like hell it doesn't.

I felt insecure, shaken, and very, very frightened. Surely this couldn't be happening. How many more bad dreams was I not going to wake up from?

By now, Mr Swann's naturally pallid complexion had become deathly white, and his arms were wrapped protectively round his midriff. I noticed beads of sweat on his upper lip. His wide-eyed look and his attempted smile resembled a bizarre grimace. He seemed more aware of the poor sound-proofing properties of the hospital curtains than Mrs Grant had appeared to be, and he must have been conscious that, as my voice increased in volume, his boss couldn't fail to hear me.

Maybe he was starting to wonder if he'd been a little hasty in telling me my operation was to be postponed. Maybe he'd only being verbalizing his hope that

Mrs Grant would opt to delay my op, and that he wouldn't be stuck in theatre until very late on a Friday evening.

The jigsaw pieces were starting to slot together in my mind. The four hour operation I'd overheard Mrs Grant discuss had indeed been my operation. My assumption that she could whip out my tumour and refashion both my breasts in a couple of hours was apparently wildly optimistic. And she'd said that she wasn't going to start it at 3pm. But surely she couldn't cancel it. I couldn't take any more disappointments and delays.

'Please calm yourself. Mrs Grant's trying her best to find a radiologist to do the localization. I'm sure she'll get one.' he whispered in an urgent voice.

I knew that Mrs Grant had a reputation for fiercely defending her patients. Mr Swann would probably get the sharp edge of her tongue if she'd heard my hysterical outburst, but frankly I didn't care. I paused, unsure about what to do, my mind racing. How could I force them to operate? What could I say to convince them? Somehow I had to persuade them.

He continued in a subdued voice, 'I'm supposed to mark you up for the operation. I'm not sure whether to or not, as we don't know whether it'll go ahead.'

I fixed him with a steady gaze. The unassuming mouse had finally scurried away. 'Let's think positively, shall we? Mark me up.'

'Marking up' means drawing on your body with a black felt-tip pen. It's done in many operations, for example, if you need a kidney removing, the doctor will draw a black cross on the correct side, as an extra fail-safe. It's just one of the many checks in place when you have an operation.

In plastic surgery, marking up can help the final cosmetic appearance. Breast surgeons who have additional onco-plastic qualifications (such as Miss Gomez and Mrs Grant) use plastic surgery techniques when a breast tumour is removed to help recreate a natural-looking breast. It's difficult to judge what the breast will look like when the patient is lying down in theatre, so the doctor plans the appearance beforehand, when the patient is standing. They make various measurements and use the felt-tip to plan where incisions will be made, and where the nipples will end up, to look natural.

'OK, can you stand up for me with your arms by your side?' Mr Swann had regained his composure. He spoke gently and politely, and with no apparent resentment at my outburst.

111

What followed was the most bizarre episode in my breast cancer experience to date.

In order to refashion my breasts, Mrs Grant would have to move the position of my nipples, because the breasts would be smaller. She would also remove every bit of breast tissue attached to my right nipple, including all the breast ducts and tiny muscle cells, to make sure there were no cancer cells left behind, and then, what was left of my nipple, just the surface, would be sewn into place at the end of the operation.

Mr Swann's job was to cover my chest in markings, to help guide Mrs Grant during all this.

He stood in front of me holding a black marker pen. He hesitated, then drew a long black line down the centre of my chest.

After this he looked at me and said, 'I have to decide where your new nipples will be now.'

He made a few measurements with a tape measure and then drew a circle for each nipple on my chest.

He didn't seem very confident. I stood there, naked to the waist, covered in black felt-tip marks, feeling completely underwhelmed.

'Are you happy with them there?' he asked.

Never having been required to decide where my nipples should go before, I didn't feel qualified to comment.

My mood was sinking into my disposable slippers. Here I was in a supposed Centre of Excellence. They couldn't even make sure there was a radiologist on duty to do my tumour localization, and now I had this dithering idiot deciding where my nipples should go. What the hell would I end up looking like? Always assuming I even had the operation.

Then, just as things seemed hopeless, the curtains parted slightly and Mrs Grant appeared in the gap.

'Is it OK if I come in?' she enquired. A somewhat rhetorical question. My eyes pleaded. She returned my look with compassion.

She took a deep breath. 'I gather you're aware of the problem. I'm trying to get Dr Frimley to do your localization. He's doing an ultrasound clinic at the moment but he says he'll do you straight after, and we'll get you to theatre as soon as he's finished.'

A warm shiver of pure relief pervaded my rigid body.

'Thank you so much, Mrs Grant. I'll make sure the nurses have me ready for

theatre so I can go straight there from the X-ray department.'

She looked at me steadily, and replied in a controlled voice,

'That's not your job. It is the nurses' responsibility to make sure you're ready.'

I wasn't sure if she was angry with the nurses, angry with me, or just angry. I didn't really care. May God bless her and all her children, she had saved my operation, and seemed prepared to go ahead even if it was a late start.

She turned her attention to Mr Swann who was standing frozen to attention, like a private unexpectedly enduring an inspection from a General.

'So, Mr Swann, I see you're marking up Dr Thompson for her operation.

'Would you like to explain to me why you've chosen those particular sites for her nipples?'

'They should be 20cm from the sternal notch' his voice was barely audible.

She looked at him for what seemed a very long time.

'Yes,' she finally replied in a quiet voice, 'you're correct. They should be twenty centimetres from the sternal notch—in a sixteen year old girl. Did you notice that Dr Thompson is not a 16 year old girl?'

I resisted the urge to show mock disappointment that she'd rumbled me as fifty plus. Definitely not the time or place, I decided.

She walked towards me, 'Do you mind if I examine you?' she spoke gently.

"No, of course not.'

Her fingers moved confidently and expertly. She examined my breasts, and made various measurements. Finally, she decided that Mr Swann's markings were absolutely fine. My confidence returned; she was making sure everything was done properly. I was going to come out of this looking OK.

As Mrs Grant disappeared through the curtains, Mr Swann raised his hand to hold them back to follow her, his head bowed and his shoulders hunched.

'Well done.' I murmured.

He started, and, closing the curtains after her, he turned to me and whispered, 'I've never seen her so angry.'

'Really? Well I'm glad I'll be fast asleep in the theatre then.' I smiled.

After they left, I decided to make sure the nurses got me ready. Time was marching on; it was already nearly one o'clock. Despite Mrs. Grant's comment that it wasn't my responsibility, I wasn't taking any chances. When the X-ray department called for me, I didn't want any further delays because I was still dressed in my day clothes. I was still hopeful that they would get me down to theatre by 2pm, my original operation slot.

I peeped out from behind the curtains. The nurses had been fairly relaxed in the morning, but now they all seemed to be extremely busy, darting between patients, in and out of side-wards. One nurse came to check I was OK. I asked her if she would get me ready for theatre, 'Yes, of course, just give me a few minutes.' She dashed off.

I sat on the trolley behind the curtains for ten minutes, but she didn't return. I decided to get dressed and draw the curtains back. At least if they saw me, they might remember I needed getting ready.

Ten minutes later I asked another nurse,

'Yes, of course, I'll be with you in a minute.'

Ten further minutes went by, and I started to pace up and down next to my bed.

'Are you OK?' called one of the nurses.

'I need to get ready for theatre before I go down to X-ray, I'm worried about the time.'

'No problem, I'll get you ready. Give me a few minutes.'

I never saw her again.

At some point during my hyperactive pacing, a handsome Italian man breezed onto the ward, wearing a stethoscope like a scarf. He stopped at my bed, 'Kathleen Thompson?'

'Yes'

'I'm the anaesthetist, can I have a quick look at you?' He was dragging the curtains around my bed as he spoke, and he attached his stethoscope to my chest in one fluid movement.

'Any health problems? Heart, lungs OK?'

'Yes, all fine.'

'Great, well I'll see you in theatre then.' He gave me a big smile and strode off the ward.

I pulled the curtains back and resumed my pacing, looking for any nurse who gave any indication of not being fully occupied.

Eventually I blocked the path of one as she hurried to the sluice, and asked her to give me a theatre gown.

'No, no, I'll get you ready, don't worry.' She stopped what she was doing and dashed to find a tape measure to size me for the anti-embolic stockings. Then she took me into a side room and asked me to jump on the scales. She jotted my weight down and then got me a theatre gown and some one-size-doesn't-fit-

anybody disposable knickers.

Theatre-ready at last, I sat, stood, paced - waiting, and waiting, for the call to X-ray.

Half of me thought calm down, it's not your problem. They have to sort this and there's nothing you can do to speed things up.

The other half of me thought they could still cancel the operation if they don't do the X-ray soon. I was sure that once they'd inserted the first wire they would have to go ahead. They couldn't possibly cancel after they'd inserted wires into my chest – that would be unethical. But until that moment, my situation felt vulnerable.

I got up and paced again, unable to sit still.

I looked at my watch for the hundredth time. It was nearly two o'clock, and I was still on the pre-op ward.

At 2.20pm, a young nurse came to my bed and smiled at me,

'You need to come with me to the X-ray department.' Her relaxed manner, and more importantly the fact that we were going to the X-ray department helped calm me.

We walked along the long corridor and into the lift down to X-ray. She spoke to the receptionist and then took me along a deserted corridor to an empty waiting room at the end.

'Someone will call you soon. I need to get back to the ward now. See you later.' She smiled brightly.

After twenty minutes had gone by, I started to worry that they'd forgotten about me. I wandered out to the reception desk.

'Hello, yes we do know you're here, someone'll call for you soon. Go back to the waiting room for now.'

I checked my watch. I didn't need to, I'd been checking it every 30 seconds for the past hour and knew exactly what time it was; it was 2.53pm and 35 seconds.

Desperate to calm myself down, I made myself relax and meditate. After a few minutes, I opened my eyes. I was definitely calmer.

At 3.05pm a young radiographer came in and, with a very serious expression, gave me a long speech about how very sorry she was that I'd had all these problems. She spoke non-stop for a long time. She was very sweet and sincere, but all I could think was yes, OK, just stop talking and let's get on with it.

Speech finished she headed out the door. I got up to follow her, but she stopped me.

'No, you need to stay here a little longer. I'm still waiting for Dr Frimley to get here. Don't worry, he's finished the clinic and he's on his way. I'm going to prepare the room for the procedure now, so when he arrives we should be able to get started. Just hang on and I'll call you as soon as he gets here.'

Another anxious twenty minutes went by before she eventually came back and took me into a small room with an X-ray machine. I went through the usual blue gown ritual, 'Put it on with the opening down the back please'. As soon as I walked into the X-ray room the nurse told me to put it on the other way round.

Dr Frimley greeted me.

'I must apologise. This was entirely the fault of our department. Because of the holidays, no-one checked that there was a radiologist on duty today. I've been stuck in the ultrasound clinic all morning, and just to make things worse, the clinic over-ran, so I've only just finished.'

'Well, thanks so much for agreeing to fill in. You poor thing, you can't have had any lunch.'

'Well, to be honest I did stop off and have a coffee and a Kit-kat on the way. I didn't think it'd help if I went hypo on you.' he gave a guilty smile.

Why was I thanking him? Why wasn't I asking him why couldn't he have come earlier and left the ultrasound patients waiting? Why had he chosen instead to risk my operation being cancelled? As he had pointed out, this whole debacle was due to his department's cock-up. He should have sorted this out sooner. Instead he'd left me in a state of acute anguish whilst he tucked into a coffee and Kit-kat. He could have drunk his coffee and eaten his damn Kit-kat as he walked along the corridor. Didn't he realize how I'd suffered, wondering where the hell he was, and exactly when was the cut-off time when Mrs Grant would phone down and tell him not to bother?

I could have asked all these things, but I just wanted him to get on and stick that first wire into my chest. So I didn't waste precious moments complaining—and bizarrely I was grateful. However unreasonable it was that I'd been put in this horrible situation, I still saw him as my saviour. Besides that, I knew that his intentions were good. He hadn't personally made the clerical error. He had his own pressures of getting through a busy clinic, and now this localization procedure had been thrust upon him. He'd responded as best he could, not even taking the time for a proper lunch break. I was also conscious from my personal experience that hospital doctors are constantly having extra work thrust upon them; it's in the nature of the job. This procedure was the most important thing

116

in my life at that moment, but for him, it was just one of a daily series of serious situations, often involving very sick patients.

But even the localization didn't go smoothly. Dr Frimley wasn't familiar with the particular X-ray machine they were using, and the radiographers didn't seem to be either. They sat me on a chair with my right breast squashed yet again between the Perspex plates of an X-ray machine for nearly half an hour, while they struggled with the machine. At one point I thought to myself, why don't they just get these wires into me and get me to theatre so I can go to sleep and get this over with? I was so tired, I hadn't eaten for many hours and I was stressed beyond all reason.

Dr Frimley must have seen the expression on my face because at that moment he said, sharply, 'Come on. We have to get this machine sorted. This poor woman needs to get to theatre.'

Finally the wires were in place, it hadn't hurt, because Dr Frimley had injected local anaesthetic first, and from their comments the procedure seemed to have been a technical success. They placed a dressing over my breast to keep the wires where they were, and called the ward nurse to take me to theatre. I breathed a very big sigh of relief. It was 4 pm, but I felt sure my operation was secured now.

The same young nurse came back and I walked with her to the lift. She was just as relaxed as before, and she ambled along slowly, chatting about everything and nothing. We waited and waited for the lift. Then she turned to me and said: 'Actually I've just remembered, the other lift would be better, it'll take us straight to theatre. Are you OK to walk a bit further?'

Well I'd walked this far hadn't I? Of course I could walk to the next lift, if it meant getting to theatre any time within the next week.

'Yes, I can walk, let's go.' I spoke quickly, hoping to inject some sense of urgency into her, but she was oblivious. She seemed to have one speed, and it was dead slow.

So we walked around to another lift, which took us straight to the basement of the hospital. The lift doors opened and I could see, at the end of a very long corridor, the theatre staff all gathered in their 'greens'. I tried to walk as quickly as I could down the long corridor as they watched us. I knew they'd been waiting for over two hours for me to arrive, and they would be willing us to hurry. The nurse was still ambling slowly along chatting. Her calm manner would have been great to relax a nervous patient in a different situation—but not this one.

'Do you think we could look like we're hurrying?' I suggested to her quietly. She *upped her pace imperceptibly.*

After what seemed an age, we reached the staff at the end of the long corridor. I recognized the friendly anaesthetist.

'I don't know where you think you're going. We're all off home.' he joked as I passed him.

I stopped dead, and whirled to face him. 'No, please don't go,' I pleaded.

'Of course we're not going home.' responded a theatre nurse, a wisp of blond hair escaping from her blue theatre cap. She gave the anaesthetist a mock scowl. 'Come through here my love, and let's get you ready.'

The anaesthetist followed us into the preparation room and, once I'd climbed onto the couch, they started to get me ready for theatre, quickly but calmly, with a constant stream of banter. I felt relaxed for the first time since Mr Swann's shock announcement. This was familiar territory for me and I slipped back into 'doctor' mode again. I joined in the banter, but like them I was also very aware of what was going on around me, and I responded immediately to their technical questions between the amusing repartee. The friendly nurse asked what job I did, 'I'm a doctor, actually.'

'Oh, I did wonder. Why didn't you say?'

'Well I think it makes people nervous.'

'Yes you're right,' the anaesthetist joined in, 'My son needed a blood test last week. When I mentioned that I was a consultant anaesthetist, the nurse asked why I hadn't said. I told her that if I had done, she'd probably have missed the vein and I'd probably have ended up having to take my son's blood myself. Just putting a cannula in, hold still for me.'

Soon the anaesthetist was starting to inject the induction agent, which would send me to sleep. As he did, I saw the theatre orderlies and nurses, quietly poised, ready to swoop in as soon as the drug took effect. I knew that in less than a minute, as soon as I was asleep, they would remove my gown and prepare my body for the operation, but as I watched the anaesthetist's hands press the plunger on the syringe I didn't care. The operation was going ahead.

What happened to me was not what you should expect on your operation day, and I'm sure my experience was quite unusual. However, things can go wrong on occasions, and people make mistakes. In my case it was a simple clerical error that had caused me such grief. I will be forever thankful for the dedication of Mrs Grant and her team, as well as the theatre staff, for starting my four hour operation after 4pm on a Friday. It meant that most of them would not leave work until nearly 9pm.

Hospital doctors don't get paid extra overtime in such situations, and I was to discover that Mrs Grant and her team worked many, many hours above their contracted quota, purely because their patients needed them. Some of the staff would be paid overtime, but they may not have chosen to work deep into a Friday night either, and yet they all appeared to do so cheerfully. I discussed this with Mrs Grant when I saw her at my out-patient appointment later. She told me that she didn't mind working late at all, but she'd been angry as she struggled to find a radiologist, because she knew how often the theatre staff ended up staying very late. It seemed she was protective not just of her patients but her staff too.

Summary:

A sentinel node biopsy will usually be taken when the breast lump is removed. If cancer is found in this node, more lymph nodes will be removed.
You may need wires inserting into your breast before your operation, to help the surgeon ensure all the tumour is removed. It is uncomfortable but not painful.
The procedure for mastectomy will be different and depends on your particular cancer.
Whatever operation you have, your surgeon will mark your breast with a felt-tip pen, to guide him during surgery.
The Informed Consent form is an important legal document. Your operation must be explained carefully to you, including any risks, and you should have time to think about it. Read the form and ask any questions you might have before you sign the form.

Further Information:

Cancer Research UK   http://goo.gl/skuHgT
Surgery (Breast Cancer Care)   http://goo.gl/Pr1xmz
American Cancer Society   http://goo.gl/RBU0t4

Operations (Breast Cancer Care)   http://goo.gl/Rtnfaa

Chapter 17

Post-operation period, complications

My Story

I opened my eyes. Everything was a swirling white mist. In the middle of the white, a spectre gradually appeared. It was Mrs Grant, smiling, her face close to mine,

'Everything went well.' The words seemed to float in the air without a source. Slowly, a vague memory of having a cancer operation registered, Ah yes. Still deeply drugged, I couldn't smile or talk. I summoned all my strength and lifted my hand to her arm and squeezed it. She smiled again, and then disappeared. Everything faded into blackness.

Some time later, I was aware of lying in bed—that snuggly feeling as sleep gently departs. Was it a work day? Could I doze for just a bit longer?

Then memories gushed in. I wasn't in bed at all. I was on a trolley in the recovery room, and I'd had my operation. I was just about to doze off again, then I remembered about the operation starting late. The theatre staff would have to stay until I was awake. I must wake up and let them go home. I summoned all my strength, opened my eyes, and started chatting.

I'm normally a quiet person, but after a general anaesthetic I turn into a rather alarming one-woman show. Soon I was entertaining the recovery staff with long tales of my skiing mishaps, explaining how to do the cha-cha-cha and detailing the finer points of western horse-riding, not to mention how to say 'Thanks, I've had enough to eat' in Chinese. They listened and smiled while they waited for the ward nurse to take me away. Someone managed to cut into my monologue to tell

121

me that my daughter was waiting.

When I arrived on the ward I saw my daughter Mickie and son Joe, my ex-husband and my friend's daughter waiting by my bed. They'd been there for hours, as I'd originally told them I would be out by 4pm. With all the uncertainty as to whether my operation would go ahead, there hadn't seemed any point in updating them until I knew what was happening, and when I finally did know what was happening, I was on my way to theatre sans mobile phone, so I hadn't warned them of the delay. It turned out that while I'd been blissfully asleep, no one had told them anything, and they had no idea when I would be coming out, or why I was so late.

It was lovely to see them and, still high on anaesthetic, I entertained them non-stop for over an hour. Eventually it occurred to me that it was very late, they were exhausted, and needed to get home.

'When do you get out, Mum?' Mickie asked.

'Tomorrow, all being well. The doctor will come to see me in the morning. Phil is going to drive me.'

'OK. Charlotte and I'll pop in to see you tomorrow. Let me know when you're home,' Joe said.

After they left, the lady from the opposite bed walked past my bed and smiled, looking puzzled. On her way back she paused then spoke, 'Have you just had an operation?'

'Yes, this afternoon.'

'Gosh, I've been on this ward for a week, and seen lots of women come back from theatre, but I've never seen anyone come back and chatter like you did. Normally they just lie there and sleep for hours.'

I grinned at her, and settled down in bed to watch television on the tiny screen attached to my bed. Eventually I did doze off, but woke repeatedly. There seemed to be an ambulance station right next to the hospital, and the sirens broke into my sleep over and over again. At 2am an alarm went off on someone's drip—a high-pitched piercing sound that went right through me. Nobody came to deal with it. It went on and on. I fumbled in the bag of presents which my friend's daughter had brought me. Where were they? Ah, here, ear plugs. Peace at last.

I didn't dare sleep too deep, because I needed my pulse and blood pressure checking throughout the night. I'd been warned that I mustn't have any blood pressure readings or blood tests from my right arm, because they'd taken the sentinel node biopsy from that side, and these procedures, together with the damaged lymph nodes, could cause lymphoedema. The charming nursing auxillary who was doing my observations kept forgetting this. I did everything I could to discourage her from using my right arm—even wheeling all the instruments and the visitor's chair around to that side so she couldn't reach my arm, but she was cheerfully persistent. Fortunately I managed to wake up every time and deflect her to my left arm.

The next morning, Saturday, Mr Swann arrived at 7am. He wore a smart striped shirt and chinos, and seemed much more relaxed. He asked me to take off my pyjama top and examined the mass of plastic and gauze dressings which swathed my chest.

'Everything looks fine, Kathleen. The operation went well. On initial look, there was no sign of tumour in your sentinel lymph nodes, so we didn't need to remove any more. Of course the pathology lab will do further tests for confirmation, but fingers crossed all will be OK.

'Now, you can shower with these dressings, but probably best to wrap cling film around them too.'

'Thanks Mr Swann. Is it OK to go home?'

'Yes, I'll get the nurses to give you an out-patient appointment.' He smiled and headed towards the nurses' station.

So, armed with a carrier bag full of spare dressings, I waited for Phil to drive me home.

Hospital stay times are getting shorter and shorter, partly to reduce patient exposure to antibiotic-resistant bacteria such as MRSA, but no doubt also to reduce NHS costs. If you are well enough, it is nice to get home as soon as possible, but you need to remember that surgery is a major stress on your body, and you need to rest and allow everything to heal. Of course, I didn't – and I paid the price.

My Story

I felt good. The dressings were wrapped so firmly around my chest that they acted like a bra. It seemed incredible that only yesterday I'd had major surgery. I didn't really know what my new breasts looked like under the bandages, but they felt OK, and actually I was quite looking forward to having smaller breasts. New boobs had not been part of my 'how to deal with middle-age' game-plan, but seeing as I'd got them I may as well enjoy them. My operation was over, the cancer had been removed, and I felt extremely happy.

When we got home, Phil made me a cup of tea and suggested I rested. I phoned my daughter and my son to let them know I was home.

After an hour or two, I fancied walking to the shops. Yes, I know a 40 minute walk involving a steep hill less than 24 hours after major surgery was not too bright an idea, but as the old expression goes, do what the doctor tells you, not what he/she does, and I was certainly not a shining example of post-operative patient conduct.

Phil came with me. He wasn't enthusiastic about my plan, but knew better than to argue. Plus, if he was honest, he'd probably have done the same thing himself. Actually I felt great sauntering down the hill and window-shopping.

On the way back, though, I started to struggle up the hill. My wounds were beginning to ache and I became breathless. I was surprised. Normally I didn't even notice the hill. I had to stop and rest, and I was glad to get back.

When I mentioned what had happened to my son later, he was less than impressed, and gave me a strong lecture on taking it easy and allowing my body to recover. It seems my kids and I were already experiencing role reversal—something I hadn't expected at a mere 55 years old.

My son was right of course, and I did try to rest after that.

Five days after my operation I went for my post-op check. As I lay on the examination couch Bronwen, the nurse, took off my dressings. I was intrigued to see the surgical handiwork for the first time. Both breasts looked good, the scars had been cleverly sited in the crease underneath them, and although long, they were not unsightly and I guessed they would fade in time.

However, my right nipple looked extremely swollen. It really didn't look healthy; maybe I shouldn't have insisted on keeping it. Was it dying?

There was a knock, and Mrs Grant's head appeared around the door,

'May I come in?' Her signature opening line.

'Yes of course Mrs Grant.'

'How are you?' she smiled.

'I'm feeling fine, thank you. Really good.'

'Let's have a look at the wounds. Oh yes, looking good. Bronwen, can you cut the dressing off the nipple?' she spoke to the petite Welsh nurse.

With that, Bronwen started snipping around my right 'nipple', and then removed it.

I realised that what I had thought was a very unhealthy-looking swollen right nipple was actually an iodine-soaked dressing. In fact, once the dressing was removed, the nipple looked fine. I breathed a huge sigh of relief.

'Oh, yes, that nipple is 'taking', Mrs Grant said. 'We have the pathology results back,' she continued, 'and they're good.' She knew better than to keep me in suspense—the full pathology assessment of the tumour was very important. She read the report out loud to me:

'A 2.5 cm area of grade 2 carcinoma, surrounded by a larger area of DCIS. The margins are clear of disease, and the sentinel lymph nodes showed no cancer.'

The clear margins meant that the edges of the removed tissue were all healthy; no cancer had been left behind.

'So that makes your breast cancer Stage 1, which is really good news.' she smiled.

Bronwen dressed the wound again and I made an appointment for two weeks' time. Things couldn't be better. I went home—and rested this time.

Twelve days after the operation, my left breast became red and swollen. Ironically, this was the breast that hadn't had the cancer. I thought it might be infected. But it wasn't too bad, maybe it would settle down. I left it three more days, by which time it was Saturday, and it was definitely worse. There wouldn't be much point phoning the hospital over the weekend, so I decided to ride it out until my next out-patient appointment on the Monday.

By Monday my left breast felt like a massive boil—red, hot and tense. I struggled into the hospital.

Mr Swann called me in, 'How are you?'

'Well, the right breast is fine, but the left one has been red and sore.'

'OK, let's take a look.'

I undressed and lay on the couch.

He examined me, 'Oh dear, it looks like you've some cellulitis.'

I felt annoyed with myself. Why had I left it? Why hadn't I sought medical help earlier? I should have known better.

Mr Swann started me on antibiotics with instructions to contact him if things didn't improve.

Two days later there was no real improvement, in fact copious amounts of pus were leaking from the wound. I was a mess of worry and guilt. After all the surgery, was my new breast going to be ruined by a deep infection? Once again, I wondered why I had been such an idiot and let it get so bad.

I made an urgent appointment to see the GP. My usual GP wasn't available. The doctor I saw looked at the wound and simply advised me to contact the hospital. I rushed home to phone, but it was already past five o'clock. Eventually, with persistence, I was put through to a male nurse. He advised me to come to the assessment ward the following morning, Thursday.

I remembered that Thursday was Mrs Grant's operating day, and Mr Swann would be scrubbed up and in theatre all day. He'd told me he wanted to know if I got worse, so I phoned Mrs Grant's secretary on the way in to ask her to tell him.

'I'm afraid Mrs Grant's team are in theatre all day. It won't be possible for any of them to come to the ward to see you.'

"But Mr Swann said I should let him know if things got worse. I really think he'll want to know.'

'Well I'll email him. That's all I can do. Sorry.'

I had a vision of Mr Swann, in his theatre greens and sterile gloves, one hand on a wound retractor, the other using a sterile keyboard to surf the internet, in the middle of a breast operation. Not very likely, was it? I sighed as I put my mobile phone back in my bag. I would just have to be insistent with the ward staff.

A young African staff nurse was at the reception desk when I got to the assessment unit. I explained that my wound infection was oozing pus, despite the antibiotics and I emphasized that Mr Swann had asked to be called when I arrived (slight poetic licence, but needs must).

'OK, come in here and I'll have a look.'

She took off my dressing and her relaxed expression turned to concern as she saw the dressing, which was saturated with pus and blood.

'When did you change this dressing?'

'This morning, about three hours ago'

'Well that is definitely pus', she dipped a swab into the wound and put it in a sterile sample container, as she spoke.

'I'll pop a little dressing on for now, then I'll let Mr Swann know you're here.'

'Thanks.'

Twenty minutes later, a young doctor walked into the room,

'Hi, Mr Swann's operating so he asked me to see you. Can I take a look?'

I undid the dressing for her.

'Oh gosh, what a lot of pus. Let me telephone Mr Swann. I'll be back in a minute.'

When she came back, she told me that he'd asked her to admit me to the ward, as I would need intravenous antibiotics.

The nurse followed her in with a drip containing the antibiotics. She put a cannula in my arm, and gave me my first dose.

'OK, these antibiotics will take about thirty minutes to go in – we need to give them slowly, for safety, as they are very strong. When they've finished you're going to Ward 5. They're expecting you.'

I sat there staring at the clear fluid dripping into my veins, willing it to do its best, still feeling angry with myself for letting things go so far.

'OK, all finished now,' the nurse was back, 'Are you alright to go to the ward by yourself or do you want someone to go with you?'

'I'll be fine thanks. It's the same ward where I had my operation, isn't it?'

'Yes, let me just put a bung in this cannula then, you'll be needing it for a few days so we should take good care of it.' She bandaged the small plastic tube sticking out of my vein.

I walked up to the ward, carrying the overnight bag I'd bought with me just in case.

A nurse showed me into a large side-ward with five beds. I took off my shoes and sat on mine and looked around at my new neighbours.

A small, bird-like middle-eastern lady was on my left. There was a woman in her thirties in the bed opposite me and a quiet middle-aged lady in the bed next to her. The fifth bed was empty.

I kept my day clothes on. It was my way of not giving in to the illness—I wanted to act and look like a 'normal' person, not a patient.

There wasn't much to do. I phoned my kids and let them know I was in hospital again, and then I let Phil know too. My antibiotics were every twelve hours, and so my next dose wasn't due until that night.

In the evening, my daughter popped in on her way home from work. She brought me some delicious chocolate covered plums, which one of her Polish workmates had recommended, and we sat and chatted.

When she left, I started to read a magazine and helped myself to one of her chocolates. I'd just put a complete chocolate plum into my mouth when I heard a familiar voice. I looked up and saw a woman smiling at me from the end of the bed. It took me a minute to register that Mrs Grant and her complete surgical team were standing around my bed. I desperately tried to give some intelligent response, but my mouth was so full of chocolate that all that came out was a mumble and a large brown dribble.

It was after 7pm, and the team must have just left the operating theatre. Another late night for them.

Mrs Grant asked if she could examine me (I wonder if anyone has ever said 'No?').

'Oh yes, the wound is certainly infected. I suggest you lie in a warm bath as often as you can, and see if you can squeeze out as much pus as possible.'

She turned to Mr Swann. 'You may need to open up the wound a little, Harry, to help the pus drain. Let's see how it goes.'

Then turning back to me she said: 'I'm so sorry this has happened'.

'Well it isn't really your fault, Mrs Grant. It can happen after any operation.'

'But I was the surgeon who operated, and I must accept responsibility' she replied. She swept out with her entourage and I hurried off to the bathroom to obey her orders.

I found the bath, but no plug. I looked for a nurse. Despite asking several nurses, no bath-plug was forthcoming, so I improvised. There was a dispenser of disposable rubber gloves in the bathroom. I discovered that if I pressed one flat into the plug-hole and turned on the taps, the pressure of the water kept it in place (Bear Grylls eat your heart out). I lay in the bath and milked as much out of my wound as I could. It amounted to about 10mls of thick pus. It was nice resting back in the warm water. Having given myself a good soap and rinse, I got dry and put on my new M&S PJs (purchased for my operation) and dressing gown, and wandered back to my bed to watch TV.

Later, the nurse came to give me my night-time dose of antibiotics. 'This'll take about 40 minutes to run through.' she said as she connected the drip up to the cannula in my arm, 'I'll come back and take it down when it's finished'.

Eventually I fell asleep.

Infection is a relatively common complication in the first week or so after any surgical operation. Bleeding is another possible complication. If anything about your wound doesn't look or feel right, or if you don't feel right, it is wise to contact your doctor—don't procrastinate like I did. If I'd started my treatment earlier, the infection would probably have cleared much more quickly. Once again, do what the doctors tell you, not what they do themselves. We are not always sensible when dealing with our own illnesses, I'm afraid.

You may encounter other problems; an operation is quite a major thing. Let me take you through some of the more common problems.

Tiredness is one. Be easy on yourself and listen to your body. It can take you quite a while to recover totally from any operation, and if you try to cheat nature by pushing yourself too soon, it will take its due one way or another, as it did with me.

Obviously pain may be a complication of surgery. Some people do suffer soreness and occasionally long-term pain problems but with modern surgery techniques and medication, it's not inevitable. If you do feel pain you should always let your doctor know. Besides the fact they may be able to help, pain may also indicate that something isn't right and that they need to look at you.

Usually your nipple will either be removed completely (options for creating a new 'nipple' have been discussed earlier) or all the small ducts and muscles below the nipple will be removed, leaving just the surface. In this case you may have permanent loss of sensation in the nipple, and your nipple will be permanently flat, and unable to become erect.

Lymphoedema is another complication of breast or underarm surgery, as discussed earlier.

A seroma is a collection of fluid, which can appear where the tumour was. It may settle by itself, but sometimes it may need to be drained.

These are the most common complications, but other things can happen occasionally too, so make sure you see your doctor early if you think anything is not quite right after your operation.

129

Summary:

Complications of surgery include infection, bleeding, pain, tiredness, numbness and lymphoedema. You may get some or none of these problems, or you may get other, rarer complications.
Do contact your doctor quickly if things don't seem right– if you leave a problem, it may be harder to treat
Do rest after your operation. You are not being lazy; your body needs to recover, and just because people get sent home rather quickly from hospitals these days doesn't mean they are fully recovered.

Further Information:

Web MD	http://goo.gl/dSmK4i
BreastCancer.org	http://goo.gl/2EHwV5
Breast Cancer Care	http://goo.gl/Rtnfaa

Chapter 18

Ward life and how to survive it

During my career I've been fortunate enough to attend various people-management training courses, and I thought I'd learned a few tricks—until I spent six days on a hospital ward. I learned far more from my fellow patients, I can tell you.

In everyday life, people may push in front of you in a queue, make you pay for more than your half of a shared meal, or take the last chocolate. It's annoying, but not life-changing. When you have cancer, or any serious illness, losing out on your share of care and attention matters more than someone swiping the toffee truffle you'd been saving for after your supper.

Cancer doesn't come with a free halo— and trust me, although my fellow patients had very serious crosses to bear, it didn't necessarily make them saints.

Let me introduce you to some of the characters who became part of my life for the next few days.

Fahima
Fahima was an elderly middle-eastern lady in the bed next to mine. We communicated mainly with smiles, and she showed me where the bathroom was when I first arrived. Her English was limited—although as I came to discover, not as limited as it appeared.

She had a stream of visitors. They were obviously a close family and their colourful interactions broke up the monotony of the ward. On that first night, her husband smiled at me as he passed my bed. He was clutching a bulging bag filled with interesting-looking pastries for her.

131

Fahima's son would visit her twice a day. As soon as he arrived, he would approach the first member of staff he saw, saying, 'I need to speak to the nurse in charge.'

Whether or not they were occupied with another patient didn't matter to Fahima's son. He was always pleasant, firm, and single-minded. What fascinated me was that the staff member would immediately leave the patient she was with and go to find the nurse in charge, who would also drop what she was doing and come straight away.

Fahima's son, standing tall and ramrod-straight, would proceed to give her a series of instructions:

'My mother needs her blood sugar testing an hour before her meal.

'I'm bringing in a special meal for her at 6 o'clock, please make sure that she has a hot drink afterwards.

'My mother needs a bath today and her hair washing.

'I've brought these yoghurts, they need to go in the fridge.'

…and on and on and on. I was amazed at the patience of the nurses. If they minded, they didn't show it.

Fahima was clearly unwell, and her son was making sure his mother got everything she needed. Nobody could criticize him for that. And he was very effective.

I deduced from her appearance and snippets I overheard from the medical staff that Fahima had advanced cancer. I felt sorry for her and her family. But she did make me smile sometimes.

She brandished her nurse call button like a TV remote control and there was a regular procession of nurses to her bedside, dealing with her many requests,

'Close window please—is cold.'

'Open window please—I need breath.'

'I lose my glasses—you have them?'

'When my daughter come?'

'TV no work.'

Every time the meal trolley appeared, before the canteen assistant had chance to serve anyone else, Fahima would shout out, 'I order Heinz mushroom soup.'

The server would search on her trolley for the soup. Not finding any, she'd wander off the ward, phone the kitchen and eventually return after 15 minutes with a bowl of soup. The rest of us eventually got our meal too.

Some of the regular staff were wise to this ploy,

'No you didn't.' replied the elderly West Indian kitchen manager, walking over to Fahima's bed and picking up the menu sheet, *'Look, your menu's still on your table, you haven't ordered anything.'*

But most of the time people seemed happy to run round in circles for her.

Angela

Angela was in the bed opposite me. Having not much to do, between my twelve hourly infusions, I couldn't help noticing her. She was probably in her mid-thirties, and I guessed that she'd had abdominal surgery very recently. She lay in bed most of the time. Occasionally she sat in her chair, her head propped up with pillows, groaning, and sometimes she'd make her way slowly and carefully to the bathroom, accompanied by one or two nurses.

Once, when I had a few hours to kill before my next lot of antibiotics, I slipped away to the small hospital garden. It was a warm sunny day and it was good to get away from the ward. I saw Angela there with her family. Her husband had pushed her in a wheelchair. I wondered what sort of cancer she had. It was strange to know that every single patient on the ward had cancer. He husband seemed a gentle, caring man. Her boys looked about 8 and 10 years old, the poor kids.

Angela's bed, like mine, had a set of electronic controls. Just by pressing a button on a handset, you could move the headrest up or down, or the foot end if you preferred. It was strange though, whenever Angela wanted her bed adjusting, she never used the bed control handset, but always reached for the nurse-call button. I couldn't really understand why, it seemed as much effort to press one control as the other, and she had to wait for a nurse to come.

Whenever a nurse passed her, she'd sigh softly. If they didn't hear, she managed to increase the volume quite markedly, until the nurse stopped whatever she was doing and went over to her.

I started to wonder if she was as weak as she appeared. I felt guilty for my uncharitable thoughts, given that she had cancer. Or at least, I did until one time when she wanted to get out of bed and into her chair. On this occasion no nurses responded to her call button. She shouted, weakly, then louder, but the nurses were busy with another patient. The next minute, after a furtive look around, she leapt quite nimbly out of bed and into her chair. Once there, after another quick look around, and she slouched weakly into her cushions.

Maureen

Maureen was in a bed on the opposite side to me, next to Angela. When I first arrived, she was semi-conscious, wearing a theatre gown and oxygen mask. She was connected to numerous monitors and a drip.

After an hour or so, she started to open her eyes and look around. She lifted her hand to her face, and in the process disconnected one of her leads. A high-pitched alarm shattered the quiet. Amy, one of the nurses came running.

'Oops, looks like you've disconnected yourself, Maureen.'

'Have I? Oh I am so sorry. Sure, I wouldn't have done that for the world, making you rush in here like that. And you being so busy an' all. I hate being a nuisance.'

'Bless you, you're not a nuisance Maureen. These leads are always getting disconnected. Now that you're awake, how're you feeling? Do you need any pain relief?'

'No, no. I'm fine. Well, I'm in a little bit of pain, but nothing to worry about. I'm fine really.'

'Well shall I get you an injection for the pain?'

'No, no need for that bother.'

'OK, let me know if the pain gets worse? This is the nurse-call button, keep it close by and press it if you need anything.'

Amy left.

Maureen looked across at me and Fahima,

'So sorry for disturbing yous.'

"Don't worry, alarms are always going off.' I replied. Fahima stared blankly. I think she was struggling with Maureen's accent.

'Where are you from?'

'Ireland.'

'Yes, I spotted that.' I smiled, 'Whereabouts?'

'Cork. Home of the Blarney stone. My husband says I must have kissed it too many times. Not that he's one to talk, he has the gift of the gab himself if anyone does.' She seemed to be speaking with effort. Her voice sounded weak.

A few minutes later Maureen started sniffling. She looked around anxiously. There was a packet of tissues on her locker. She reached for it. As she stretched, I saw her wince. She fell back, beads of sweat on her forehead. She waited a minute, breathing heavily, then tried again to reach the tissues, her nurse-call button lying untouched by her side. I wanted to help her, but I was attached to my antibiotic drip and couldn't move from my bed.

'Maureen, be careful, you should call the nurse.'

But my warning was too late. In her second unsuccessful attempt to launch herself at the tissues, she'd once again set off an alarm. This time her pulse monitor was loudly warning that her heart rate had gone into super-drive.

Amy rushed back in, 'Maureen, are you OK? You're very pale and clammy.'

'Oh my God, I'm so sorry. I'm being a right nuisance, so I am. I just needed a tissue and the alarm went off.'

'Listen, Maureen, you need to lie quietly for at least four hours after your operation. If you need tissues, please call me.'

'I can't call you just to pass me a tissue.' Maureen started to laugh, then immediately winced again and clutched her stomach.

'Yes you can, and you must Maureen. I'd rather pass you a tissue than pick you up off the floor when you collapse. Promise me now?'

Maureen gave a non-committal smile.

'Now I noticed you flinched when you moved. Are you sure you don't want any pain relief?'

'Ehm, well maybe while you're here, could I trouble you for a wee painkiller— maybe a paracetamol or something?'

'Of course Maureen, but you need more than paracetamol. I'll pop and get you an injection.'

I looked at my watch. It was 2am. Angela and Fahima were gently snoring. Maureen was moaning quietly. She sounded like she was in a lot of pain. The night nurse gave her an injection and changed her drip bag at around 3am, then left, forgetting to turn her light off. I watched as Maureen held her hand up to shade the light from her eyes and I could see her puzzling over the bed controls. After a while she seemed to give up, dropped the controls and, reaching for her small hand towel, draped it over the light. The next day, I showed her where the light switch was on her bed control. I knew she would never bother the nurses, and I was worried we'd all go up in flames if she tried the towel trick again.

Two days later Maureen was starting to walk around, slowly and carefully, but always with a bright 'I'm fine and not in pain at all' smile.

At midday I lay attached to my antibiotic drip and watched as she made her way to the bathroom, wheeling a drip stand in her right hand and clutching her stomach with her left, fingers splayed and tense, as if she was trying to prevent her stomach contents from bursting through the front of her nightie.

As she passed Angela's bed, Angela looked up from her magazine and gave a loud moan as if in severe pain.

I returned to my book, becoming gradually aware that I needed to go to the loo. I looked up at the bag of antibiotics, gradually emptying. There was still fluid in there. I crossed my legs and willed it to finish.

Fifteen minutes later, the bag was empty. I was pretty desperate now, my bladder felt like an overfilled balloon and I was getting cold sweats. Please let Nurse Amy come quickly to disconnect me.

As I waited, legs firmly clamped, I became aware that the hospital chaplain, who'd been having a few words with Angela, was heading my way.

Oh no, please not now.

'Hello dear, how are you? I don't think we've met.' She took my hand.

'Fine thanks.'

'So how long are you in here for?'

'Not sure.' I was anxiously looking past her for any evidence of Amy's rescue.

'Well I'm the hospital chaplain. Do you have a religion?'

'RC.' I was getting really desperate now. My breathing was getting fast and I was screwing up my pelvic muscles like a Pilates fanatic. I even considered pressing the nurse call button. Where was Amy?

'Really? Well I'm C of E. We have a number of chaplains who cover here. We do a rota, but if you want to speak to a Roman Catholic priest I could call him.'

'No, really, it's fine. I'm fine. I'm just waiting for the nurse. Ah, Amy, my infusion's finished,' I called as Amy turned the corner.

'Ah yes, well OK dear. It's been nice talking to you.' The chaplain smiled, but I noticed a slight look of reproach in her eyes.

'Nice talking to you too,' I called after her. She was a really sweet person, I felt so mean. She must have thought me so rude, but I was desperate.

'OK, let's release you. Everything OK?' Amy started unscrewing the drip from my cannula.

'Yes fine. Listen, I'm desperate for the loo, Amy. I need to dash.'

I nearly bowled the poor chaplain over as I dashed past her and around the corner to the bathroom. I burst open the bathroom door, and nearly somersaulted over a large bottom blocking my path.

'Maureen? What are you doing?'

Maureen was bent over, wiping the floor with a heavily bloodstained towel.

'I've started bleeding and made such a mess.'

'Maureen, you can't clean this up yourself.' Before she could stop me, my hand darted past her and yanked the red nurse-call cord.

'Oh, you didn't need to do that.'

'Yes I did, you're looking really shaky, and I'm sorry but I'm bursting for the loo.'

'What's going on here?'

I breathed a sigh of relief, and gave my pelvic floor muscles one last tweak as I heard Amy's squeaky flats heading towards the bathroom.

'Maureen, you terror, what have I told you?' Amy guided Maureen into a wheelchair, unhooked the bag of fluid from the drip stand, and holding it high in her right hand she wheeled Maureen back towards her bed using just her left hand and right elbow.

The second they were through the door, I slammed it shut, pulled down my drawers and plonked myself down on the loo.

The relief was heavenly.

Angela and Fahima instinctively knew how to work the hospital system. I have no idea what was going on in Angela's life that made her crave attention. The woman had young sons and cancer—who knew what her outlook was? But the pie of nursing attention is only so big, and if some people help themselves to an unnecessarily large slice, there may only be diet portions left for others.

Maureen and I fell into the 'put on a brave face, do what you can for yourself and don't complain or demand' camp—not always a successful strategy when you're sick. In Maureen's case, I believe she actually made Amy's job harder by trying to be independent, and she certainly took risks by not asking for help when she should have done. However, I could understand her reluctance, I (and many others) feel it too.

The trouble is, nursing is called the 'caring profession' for a reason—and nurses are 'programmed' to help sick people; it is their raison d'etre, and they are human beings. Some nurses find it hard to deal with patients who seem too independent, who appear not to need or want help, whereas patients such as Angela press all the right buttons (including the nurse-call button), making their carers feel needed, and are rewarded with lots of attention. I'm not saying what is right or wrong, but it is important to be aware of the effect you are having on people and what the likely response will be—and hospital is quite a unique ecosphere if you're not used to it. People don't always reward you for being too undemanding.

Just as patients vary in their approach to illness and hospital care, so do the carers themselves. Let me tell you about some of the staff I met during my stay.

Nurse Amy

Mid-twenties, dark and petite, Amy was quiet but efficient. On the first morning after my admission, she appeared with my tamoxifen tablet, and asked me about my infected wound.

'I'll come along about ten-ish to dress it for you.' 'Your antibiotics are quite powerful, so we need to monitor your blood levels to keep them out of the toxic range. I'll check them today, then we can adjust the dose if needed. For the same reason, it's really important you have them as close to twelve hours apart as possible so the blood levels stay as steady as possible. That way we know they're always high enough to kill the bugs, but not high enough to harm you.

'I see you're dressed. If you feel like having a wander around the hospital until ten, then just let me know when you leave the ward. It's a bit boring sitting around all day isn't it?'

After she'd gone, I went for a walk. I popped into the little WRVS shop and then went and sat in the small garden. I made sure I was back on the ward for ten o'clock for my dressing. Then I had another wander around before going back to my bed in plenty of time for my mid-day antibiotics.

As Amy set up the drip, we had a chat, 'How long have you worked here, Amy?'

'Oh I'm not full time here —I just do a couple of agency shifts each week. My main job is as a research nurse at one of the other cancer hospitals—which I love. It's fascinating being involved with the latest research. When you see some of the patients, it really gives me a buzz to think we're helping them.'

As she spoke, she allowed the clear liquid to work its way down the tubing. When it started to drip out of the end, and onto her gloved fingers, she rolled the small white plastic valve to stop the flow.

I watched her picking at the sticky tape covering the cannula in my arm, 'I know what you mean,' I said. 'I work in research too, for pharmaceutical companies. If you're working on a drug for a nasty condition it can be so rewarding—particularly when patients write to you, just to tell you what a difference your treatment has made.

'I suppose you need to do agency work to supplement your income?'

She unscrewed the cap from the cannula in my arm and connected the end of the tubing to it, 'Actually it isn't the pay. I do agency because I don't want to get rusty at ward work. Keep my hand in, y'know. Besides I really enjoy it.' she taped the tubing in place, 'OK, you're stuck here for 45 minutes now. We have to give this really slowly. When it's finished I'll come and take it down for you. Next dose will be midnight. Sorry it's not very sociable, but they needs to be exactly 12 hours apart.'

'Oh, that's fine. I'll probably be asleep when the next one goes up.'

Monique

One of the cleaners, Monique, would stand and chat sympathetically to Angela, leaning on her sweeping brush—for most of her shift, actually. Angela appeared to enjoy the attention. In contrast Monique was quite offhand with me, not that I was particularly bothered.

Two days after my admission, Mr Swann made his daily visit to see me.

'How's the wound today?'

'Well, I'm still squeezing a lot of pus from it every time I get in the bath.'

'Let's take a look.' He pulled the curtains around as I undressed.

'Hmm, I think I should open it up a little, make the hole larger, allow the pus to drain. Don't worry, it won't hurt, the nerves to your skin were cut during the operation.'

He disappeared behind the curtains and returned a few minutes later with a dressing pack. He should probably have asked a nurse to come and help him, but he struggled to do everything himself—rather like me.

As he came back through the curtain, I noticed Monique just outside, with her sweeping brush.

I could see her brush below the curtain. It wasn't moving very actively, in fact, she seemed to be sweeping the same small area – just next to my curtain.

As Mr Swann's scalpel sunk into my infected wound, pus poured out, covering my chest, and the sterile towel where he'd put his instruments.

'Crikey!' he cried out, 'that's a huge amount of pus! I didn't realize just how much there was in there.'

The sweeping brush beneath the curtain suddenly froze. I noticed a gradual bulge appear in the curtain, directly above the brush, at about the height of

Monique's head.

'*Let's try and get as much of it out as possible,*' *Mr Swann gently squeezed the wound edges as he spoke.*

'*I'll take a swab, just in case we need to change your antibiotics. That must have been pretty painful for you.*' *He stared at me with deep sympathy.*

Monique treated me with a new respect from that point onwards.

Nurse Christine

Christine was a petite, attractive staff nurse with curly auburn hair. She looked after me on the third day—sort of. She came and introduced herself after the morning handover.

At 11.50 am I made sure that I was on my bed. I didn't want to keep her waiting when she came with my antibiotics.

By half past twelve there was no sign of her, and I was becoming anxious.

I couldn't see any nurses around. I stared at the nurse call button as if it was a live electric wire. Dare I press it? Maybe it would it annoy some harassed nurse, who'd been doing something terribly important with another patient? Eventually, Fahima saved the day. She pressed her call button because she couldn't find her tissues, so I was able to catch Christine on her way back from Fahima.

'*Excuse me, sorry to bother you Christine,*' *I called,* '*I know you're busy, but I was wondering when I was going to have my 12 o'clock antibiotics?*'

'*Oh? Oh, yes, your antibiotics. Umm, yes, they're next on my list.*' *With that she walked off dreamily, staring out of the window, and sniffing at some flowers in a vase as she went.*

I waited and waited. I was mentally going through what she would need to do to prepare the antibiotics—get drug cupboard keys, check drugs with another nurse, wash hands, mix water with antibiotic powder, draw the mixture into a syringe, syringe it into the bag of saline, write the label, attach the tubing, run the drug through to the end of the tubing. I went through this mental process four times, each time trying to pause for as long as I estimated the task would take. Still no sign of her. What was keeping her? It was nearly one o'clock. Amy had stressed how important it was that my antibiotics were given on time.

Another nurse was giving out some drugs to the ladies opposite. Then Christine walked onto the ward – thank Goodness, at last.

She had her handbag over her arm. She didn't look at me, but went straight over to the other nurse, '*Hi, I'm off for lunch now. See you in an hour*'.

I shouted to her, 'Christine, what about my antibiotics?'

A look of surprise, followed by recall and then annoyance crossed her face—but only briefly, 'Oh yes, your antibiotics. I'll ask a colleague to give them to you...' and she was off to lunch. By the time I got my antibiotics they were nearly two hours late.

Maybe Christine had been busy, and maybe there was an important reason why she had to go to lunch immediately. Maybe, but I was under her 'care' again the following day, and exactly the same thing happened. Once again I had to call after her as she disappeared off to lunch, and once again she palmed me off on a colleague, very late.

Amy had given me my tamoxifen tablet on my first morning in hospital, and I knew the nurses checked what drugs patients were due and gave them routinely. So I fully expected Christine to bring me my tamoxifen at some point during the following morning too. I'd always taken it religiously at home—after all it was to prevent my cancer returning—but it wasn't until that evening that I suddenly realised she hadn't brought it. Feeling sick with worry and frustration, I rushed to find her. She was in the small treatment room.

'Christine, I didn't get my tamoxifen this morning.'

'Oh? Does it matter?' she stared at me blankly, as if I'd mentioned that she'd forgotten to buy the Pope a birthday card, and continued to stack piles of sterile gauze packs onto a shelf.

'Well they are to prevent my cancer returning, so yes it does.'

She glanced up at the ward clock, then strolled over to the drug trolley and picked out my prescription card from the folder. Slowly she checked my medications, then unlocked the drug trolley and hunted around for the tamoxifen, took a tablet out and, without speaking, handed it to me.

On the fifth day, Mr Swann came back to see the wound. He was pleased with progress.

'Come down to the clinic tomorrow, about 10 o'clock. If it looks OK then, you may be able to go home. Mrs Grant'll be in the clinic, so I can always get her to take a look if need be.'

I was excited when I went to bed that night—potentially my last night. The only slight shadow was that Christine was back from her day off, and she was on nights.

She walked around all the patients at the start of her shift. When she got to me,

141

I decided I had to address my concerns, 'Hello Christine, did you have a good day off?'

'Oh yes thanks, brilliant. It was great to be away from the ward. Such a pain to be back at work.' She picked up the observation chart at the bottom of my bed, as she told me all about her day off. She seemed more animated than I'd ever seen her. After she'd finished talking she put the observation chart back and wandered off towards Fahima's bed.

'Christine, before you go, I wanted to mention that my antibiotics are due at midnight tonight.'

'Yes? Are they?' she continued moving towards Fahima as she spoke.

'Yes, and you remember that it's really important that these antibiotics are given on time? So, Christine, who will be giving me the antibiotics tonight?'

'Oh, I will.'

'And you'll be able to give them on time?'

'Yes, of course.'

Well, at least I'd got a commitment from her. I vaguely remembered from some management training course that this was a good idea. So what should I do? I tended to fall asleep around 10 o'clock—the infection had left me fairly drained. Should I let myself sleep and trust Christine to give the antibiotics, as all the other night staff had done? Or should I force myself to stay awake just in case she forgot again? Her track record had been 100% unreliable so far, but she'd promised me specifically that she would give them to me on time.

I lay there dozing, but in the end, I just couldn't risk it, I had to stay awake. Around 11pm, Fahima had problems. I wasn't sure what was wrong, but Christine and the other nurse were going back and forward to her bed, and it seemed pretty serious. Around ten minutes to midnight things had settled down. All was quiet. I waited for Christine. Midnight passed, no Christine. Thirty minutes later I pressed the scary nurse call button.

'Oh, Hi. What's wrong?'

'Christine, My antibiotics were due at midnight.'

'Oh, OK. I'll do them shortly.'

She disappeared into the other part of the ward.

At 1am she passed me en route to see Fahima. I caught her on her way back, 'Christine?'

'Oh yes, your antibiotics, I'll ask a colleague to do them.'

At 1.30am I eventually had my antibiotics.

Christine had never actually given them to me herself, and I began to wonder if she knew how.

Nurse Bronwen

The next morning at 9.45am I left the ward, walked down the modern steel staircase and headed for outpatients.

'It's looking much better,' Mr Swann commented as Bronwen cleaned the wound and changed the dressing.

'There's a deep hole there, which'll take a couple of months to heal, so you'll need to keep packing the wound until it closes up,' he continued.

Bronwen looked up from her task, 'Are you OK changing the dressing yourself? If not, your GP can organize a nurse to do it for you.'

'I can do it myself, if you could just show me, Bronwen.'

'Of course I'll show you. So we need to get right down to the bottom of this hole.' She gently pushed the gauze deep into the gaping wound in my breast, using sterile forceps. 'Then, once you have it as clean as possible using this sterile water, take some fresh gauze and pack it into the wound. Pack it fairly snugly, but not too tight, or the wound won't have a chance to close up.

'Let me give you all the dressing stuff, then you're good to go. Change the dressing every other day, and give me a call if you run into problems.' she patted my arm.

She filled a carrier bag with various special dressings, sterile saline, sterile dressing packs, sterile forceps and alcohol wipes until it was bulging, and handed it to me.

'Thanks, I'll be prepared if civil war breaks out on my way home with this lot' I joked.

'When are you going for your radiotherapy appointment?' she asked.

'I'm seeing Dr Peters next week.'

'OK, book an appointment to see me on the same day, just beforehand, and I can check your wound and change your dressing. They'll tell you at the desk that the clinic's full, but just explain that you're seeing me, and they'll squeeze you in.'

Bronwen was a lively, bright but unassuming person. Over the ensuing weeks I was to learn why she was head of the out-patient department. Like Eileen, she had that uncanny knack of treating every patient as if they were the only person she had to deal with. She was clearly extremely busy all the time, and yet she always worked my many visits for wound dressings around my schedule, not hers. Whenever she could she arranged them around my other hospital visits so I wouldn't need to make extra trips.

She always gave me her personal attention, when she could just as easily have asked one of her nurses to dress my wound. I knew she was always at the end of a phone if I needed help. She also held the position of radiotherapy nurse, and when I started my radiotherapy treatment, she drip-fed me the information I needed on what would happen to my body during the process. She knew from experience exactly what to tell me and when. Not too soon that I wouldn't be able to take in the information, but usually a few days before I realised I needed to know it. She smoothed my path through the whole anxious time.

I walked back to the ward with new-found energy and a big beam decorating my face. Although most of the ward staff had been great, I was starting to get stir crazy, and I was longing for home.

'Ah, there you are, we need to check your blood levels today.' the staff nurse greeted me as I walked back onto the ward.

'No, you don't. I'm going home. Mr Swann said I don't need any more antibiotics.'

'Oh that's lovely news,' she smiled. Do you need dressings to take home?'

'No thanks, Bronwen gave me loads.'

'I might have known. Right, well, will someone be coming to pick you up?

'My friend's meeting me outside—she'll take me home' I lied. I didn't want any more hold-ups, and I was happy to go home on the train by myself.

'OK, that's great. Let me just take your cannula out and you can go when you're ready. Have you got an outpatient appointment?'

Most of the care I received was excellent, but in healthcare, one individual not doing their job properly can be serious. What do you do if this happens? Or better still, how do you avoid the situation? It became apparent to me that the more demanding patients not only got more attention, but the staff didn't seem to mind their demands either. Even Christine would devote hours to helping Fahima, while she made no effort to remember to give me my medication. So, a few tips:

1. Politely but firmly request what you need in an audible voice and without apology. No 'I'm really sorry to bother you...' this just gives the message that

you are not important and nor are your needs. Just changing your attitude to your own self-worth tends to influence other people's reaction to you, not just in the hospital, but in life.

2. If, despite this, someone is still not giving you the care you need and should expect, ask to speak to their senior. There is always a nurse on the ward designated as Nurse-in-charge. In the case of other healthcare workers or junior doctors, you can ask to speak to your consultant. People may or may not feel antagonized by this, but at the end of the day, it's your health that's at stake. They will tend to try hard to make sure you're satisfied so that you don't complain again. But if they regard you as uncomplaining, you're more likely to be overlooked, particularly if others are demanding. It's not personal, just human nature.

3. Make your demands early, not after sitting in worried silence for an hour or three. No one will thank you for keeping your worries to yourself, and if you raise your profile, more people will consider your needs. If you fade into your hospital bed counterpane, then, when they're busy, you may slip their mind altogether.

4. If things really deteriorate, or gross misconduct is involved, there are official complaint routes, as discussed elsewhere in this book, but it's far better for everyone if things can be resolved before this point.

Remember also that most people, particularly in the healthcare profession, want to do their best. Sometimes they have genuine pressures of which you're not aware, such as seriously ill patients elsewhere in the hospital, and they genuinely have to prioritise for urgency and clinical need. Just reminding them of your needs in a firm but non-confrontational way may be all that's required.

I agonized about what I should do about Christine. Other than a minor grumble to one of the night nurses, I hadn't complained—but what about other patients she may be dealing with, who were less able to ask for what they needed? In the end, a few weeks after I left hospital, I received a patient satisfaction questionnaire. It had a section for comments. Without naming names, I made suggestions that would address the problems I'd had with Christine—such as reinstating a formal drugs round so that every patient's drug needs are regularly checked. I'm not saying this was the best approach to alerting the hospital about inadequacies in care – but it's what I did.

Summary:

Some patients will demand most of the nurses' attention –in some cases this is justified, sometimes not. Be prepared to make sure you get the care you need too. Tips to help:

- Politely but firmly request what you need, audibly and without apology.
- Your attitude can influence people's reaction to you.
- If needed, ask to speak to someone more senior, eg, Nurse-in-charge or your consultant.
- Even if people resent your complaint, they will try to stop further complaints.
- Uncomplaining patients are more likely to be overlooked – this is human nature.
- Ask for help without delay
- Remember that most people, particularly healthcare workers, want to do their best.

Further Information:

Book: The Breast Cancer Book by V. Sampson and D Fenlon, Vermilion, 2000

Chapter 19

Chemotherapy

You may need chemotherapy during your breast cancer treatment. I didn't, so I have no personal experience to share with you here.

Chemotherapy involves powerful drugs called cytotoxics (meaning toxic to cells). They are capable of damaging cancer cells, but can damage healthy cells too. Not surprisingly, this can result in side-effects. By careful dosing regimes, the aim is to destroy as many cancer cells as possible, while allowing normal cells to recover.

Different cytotoxic drugs have different side-effects, and some are more effective than others in certain cancers. Your specialist will choose the drugs and the dosing regime to treat your particular cancer type best.

Some drugs are designed to home in on a certain part of the body in order to target a particular cancer. For example special molecules called antibodies can be attached to the drug, and these take it directly to the cancer. Herceptin is a drug that can specifically target some types of breast cancer. Sometimes it can affect the heart, and if you need Herceptin your doctor will talk to you about this.

Cytotoxic drugs are often given in cycles, so you may receive several courses of treatment. This allows your healthy cells to recover in between cycles. In breast cancer, it's usually given as short courses of treatment, every two to four weeks, over a four to six month period. Medical research is always striving to optimize chemotherapy regimes though, and so approaches to treatment continually change.

Whether or not you are offered chemotherapy depends on various factors: your type of cancer, the size of the tumour, and whether it's spread elsewhere in the body, as examples. A common place for breast cancer to spread first is the lymph nodes under your arm. That's why your doctor is keen to know whether these nodes are clear of cancer. If cancer is found there, it doesn't necessarily mean the cancer has gone anywhere else; one of the purposes of lymph nodes is to capture cancer cells, and infection too, and prevent either from spreading within the body.

However, if cancer cells are found in a lymph node, it does mean that the cancer has gone beyond your breast, and sometimes cancer breaks through the lymph node defences and spreads further, so generally if the cancer has reached the lymph nodes you will be offered chemotherapy.

Usually you will receive chemotherapy after your surgery, but sometimes you'll have it beforehand, to reduce the size of your tumour before your operation.

Sometimes the intention is to give you chemotherapy to cure your cancer. Sometimes, if the cancer is more advanced, 'cure' may be unlikely, however it can still help significantly, by reducing the size of your cancer.

If you're not clear why you need chemotherapy, do ask your doctor or your Breast Care Nurse—it's important that you understand, and the reason may not be as bad as you are imagining.

Chemotherapy is undoubtedly a powerful treatment. Some people sail through it with few problems, carrying on with their work between their treatments. Others find it tough. We all react differently to cancer treatments, both physically and psychologically. It's just the way it is, and it's no reflection on individuals, so please listen to your own body and be kind to yourself.

You may experience side-effects during treatment, such as gastro-intestinal problems (nausea/sickness/sore mouth/diarrhea), fatigue and/or hair loss. In addition, your blood components can be affected, making you more prone to infection or bleeding. This will be monitored carefully and your treatment may need to be reduced or slowed down to allow the blood cells to recover.

You may suffer from hair loss—not just on your head, but eyebrows, eyelashes and body hair too. This depends on the particular drugs and sometimes your response to them, so don't assume this will happen. Check with your doctor or nurse. There are various techniques, which can help minimise hair loss, such as wearing a special hat to keep the scalp very cold during treatment sessions. This reduces the blood flow, and hence the amount of drug reaching the hair follicles.

148

Naturally you may be distressed at this prospect. It is possible to make yourself feel glamorous though. There is an excellent charity called Look Good Feel Better, which offers a free workshop to teach women with cancer how to use makeup most effectively—partly to hide or minimize the effects of hair loss and other effects of cancer treatment, but also just to help them look good and feel better about themselves during such a difficult time—and why not? There are also some useful YouTube videos, including the Baldly Beautiful ones, from a fabulous lady who took time out during her own chemotherapy to help others with their makeup (see link below). This young woman really proves how the right makeup, know-how and accessories can have a dramatic effect on your appearance.

Despite the popular image of cancer sufferers losing weight and looking frail and waif-like, this isn't always the case. In fact, breast cancer chemotherapy can cause weight gain, partly due to the steroids—which are frequently prescribed —and sometimes due to nibbling sweet things to combat the nausea. Life really is a bitch. This can be yet another blow to your self-confidence at a time when you least need it.

Chemotherapy can bring on the menopause and in younger women affect fertility. You should discuss this with your doctor before you start treatment if you are planning to have children. Various options, such as harvesting your eggs for future use may be an option. Again, this all depends very much on your individual case and what treatment you will actually receive, so please don't panic. Talk to your doctor and see whether it's likely to be a problem first.

In addition to the physical effects, chemotherapy can affect you psychologically. I've already mentioned the psychological effects of hair loss and weight gain, but the simple fact of having chemotherapy itself can have a huge effect mentally.

The word 'Chemotherapy' strikes as much fear into people's hearts as the word 'Cancer'. It creates an instant image of someone looking pale, sick, wearing a scarf on their bald head and permanently accompanied by a rather quiet chap dressed in a long black hooded gown and carrying a large garden implement with a sharp curved blade at the end.

You can hear a thousand times that chemotherapy has improved over the years, or that cancer is being detected earlier, and many people can and do survive treatment. Nevertheless, our long-held perceptions are etched into our psyches. So of course we're going to be a little shaken when we find that we've got our own front-row seat at the Chemo Concert, and audience participation is required.

First, it's sometimes best to acknowledge your fear. It's natural and it's there. You don't always have to put on a brave face. People work in different ways, and some need to deny that they feel frightened, or even deny they have breast cancer, and that's OK too. Denial can sometimes be quite a successful strategy.

However for many, it's good to express your feelings and fears. Who you choose to off-load to depends on your needs and available options, your partner, family, friends or healthcare professionals, which can include your GP, your cancer specialist, your Breast Care Nurse or a professional counsellor. Some people prefer patient support groups or on-line forums, such as those run by Breast Cancer Care. Cognitive Behavioural Therapy (CBT) is a counselling technique which can be helpful in this situation, and is available on the NHS.

As I said, I didn't need chemotherapy, but I have friends who went through it, came out the other side and are now back leading full and normal lives. Take courage, you can get through it too.

Summary:

Cytotoxic drugs can damage both cancer cells and healthy ones.
Chemotherapy is often given as several courses of treatment to allow healthy cells to recover in between.
You may need chemotherapy, depending on the type and size of the tumour, and whether it has spread outside the breast.
You may experience side-effects such as stomach problems, tiredness, bleeding, infections or hair loss.
Fertility may be affected and should be discussed if you are planning to have children later.
You may suffer psychologically, and benefit from professional help for this.
A great deal can be done to help with the cosmetic effects of chemotherapy.

Further Information:

Breast Cancer Care	http://goo.gl/wucnzh
Breast Cancer Care (Side Effects)	http://goo.gl/ZVOAUm
Look Good Feel Better	http://goo.gl/uEq4Wa
Baldy Beautiful Tutorials	http://goo.gl/fyIRLV
Breast Cancer Care Community	http://goo.gl/m11F0i
BreastCancer.org	http://goo.gl/HyX0PR
NHS Choices	http://bit.ly/1GCoqq5

Chapter 20

Radiotherapy

Radiotherapy can damage and destroy all cells, if the dose is high enough. Cancer cells are more sensitive than normal ones, and because the radiation beams are usually directed from two or more different angles, overlapping at the tumour site, the cancer also gets a higher dose than surrounding normal tissue. Hence, the plan is to destroy the cancer whilst limiting damage to your normal tissues.

After my operation, I was given three weeks of radiotherapy to the whole breast, followed by a further week just to where the lump had been (called a boost), which at the time of writing is fairly standard treatment. In the past, the course would have been longer, but studies have shown that four weeks is just as effective in many situations. Treatment regimes are constantly being improved through research. For example, doctors are currently testing whether they can give the radiotherapy internally at the time of the operation. If it works, it would represent another improvement, as it would eliminate the need for daily treatments, and reduce the overall dose of radiation too.

At the moment though, the radiation is usually given as X-ray beams. The dose, and what direction the rays should take, is carefully planned, so that the area which needs treating receives the biggest dose.

Radiotherapy is usually given either to treat the cancer, or to prevent it coming back. Sometimes it will be given before the breast operation, but more usually it will take place after both surgery and any chemotherapy are finished. The sessions are five days a week, with weekends off for good, bad or any other kind of behaviour in which you choose to indulge.

People's reaction to radiotherapy varies. Some people breeze through it, others struggle. There are many reasons why: the actual dose of radiotherapy you need, your state of mind and your physical state will influence the way you react.

I won't lie, I dreaded it and just longed for it to be over. My mother had needed it before she died, and I was beginning to share her fear of those unseen rays. But that was just my reaction; you may not find it a problem.

First you'll meet your radiotherapist—a doctor who specializes in this area. They'll explain all about the particular regime they're planning for you and any side-effects you may experience.

So what side-effects are likely?

During the first few treatments, you probably won't feel different or notice any change. Then, after a couple of weeks, your skin will usually start to go red, like sunburn, over the area where the radiation beam passes through it. As the waves go in straight lines, your radiotherapy redness will have straight edges—and this, coupled with the fact that it's concentrated on your breast, gives it a bizarre appearance, as if you'd been sunbathing in a very odd, and rather inappropriate, swimming costume.

Sometimes your skin will become permanently dark, although often, once the redness settles, it returns to a normal colour. Much later, small broken veins may appear over the area.

Your breast may become swollen and uncomfortable during treatment. Later fibrosis can occur, which may make your breast shrink (a little, or sometimes more) and become firm. Sometimes the affected breast may swell afterwards, due to lymphedema, which may also affect your arm. This is usually if the lymph nodes in your armpit have also been treated.

You may feel tired during treatment or afterwards. Some people notice no more effect than if they were popping to the shops. Others feel completely knocked out. Tiredness can increase over time, and can last for months afterwards. Radiotherapy affects your cells for longer than the duration of the treatment, and the emotional effect can also linger. As the cancer cells are damaged and broken down, the body has to deal with the inflammation, and this can reduce your energy. Going to the hospital five days a week for four weeks can contribute too, and there's the psychological impact. Some people find having radiotherapy frightening. This all adds to the stress and tiredness.

Very rarely, your lungs and/or (in the case of cancer of the left breast) your heart, may suffer some long-term damage, but this is unusual nowadays. You may get stiffness in the shoulders, and it's important to keep moving your shoulder through its full range of movement, even after your treatment has finished.

You may feel temporary, or sometimes permanent, pain and tenderness. On rare occasions the radiation can weaken bones in the area—ribs usually— sometimes causing fractures, or damage the nerves in your armpit, which can affect sensation and movement in your arm.

Your radiotherapist should also explain very carefully about the potential benefits to you of treatment. This is important, as some people will get more from radiotherapy than others, depending on their age, the size and type of tumour and other factors. Usually, if radiotherapy is offered, the upside is worth the discomfort and any long-term consequences. However, sometimes the gain is relatively small—for example, if you were already in a low risk group. In this case, you may or may not decide it's worth going through the treatment. It's a very personal decision, but you do need to understand the specific benefit for your particular circumstances in order to make an informed decision.

A word of caution: if your radiotherapist quotes statistics, make sure you get them to explain exactly what these mean. For example, if your particular cancer has a 90% chance of 'cure' after surgery alone, and radiotherapy improves the figure to 95%, this means radiotherapy will increase your chance of 'cure' by 5%. Another way of looking at it would be to say that your risk of the cancer coming back has decreased from 10% to 5%. It is exactly the same.

However 5% is half of 10%—so you could also say your risk of cancer coming back is *halved*. Put this way, the benefit seems far greater than improving survival from 90% to 95%, although it is exactly the same.

In contrast, someone else may have a worse outlook—say a 20% risk of the tumour coming back with, and 40% without, radiotherapy. That is also a halving, but a decrease in potential cancer recurrence from 40% to 20% would seem much more worthwhile than in the first example.

Unfortunately there are quite a few ways of describing cancer treatment benefits, so make sure you really understand, and don't be afraid to ask and ask again until you're sure.

I emphasise this because it's important that you make an informed choice. To be honest, I didn't at the time. I didn't do any research, and it wasn't explained in detail to me. I just trusted that I would be given the best treatment. Most of the time you will be, but people's opinion on what is an acceptable risk and what are acceptable side-effects differ. Only by completely understanding what is at stake can you make the decision best suited to you.

My Story

Bronwen carefully removed the dressings from my infected wound, 'So Kathleen,' she said, 'it's about a week since you went home from the ward, isn't it?'

'Yes, almost a week.' I replied.

'Have you been managing to clean it OK?'

'Yes, it's still oozing a bit, but that special dressing you gave me helps.'

'Oh, the alginate? I may try something else today—something a bit more absorbent, so you can leave it a bit longer between dressings. That'll give the wound a chance to heal.'

She put the final plaster on and gave me a bag of new dressings.

'Right, so you're off to see Dr Peters now? When he gives you a date for your Planning CAT scan, pop back to out-patients and book in at the same time for me to check your dressing.'

'Thanks Bronwen, that's really helpful.'

I left the outpatients and went in search of the radiotherapy department. There didn't seem to be any signs. Radiotherapy departments are sometimes a bit like nuclear bomb shelters—everyone knows they exist, but no one's quite sure where they are.

Eventually after asking a few porters, I discovered a narrow staircase, hidden behind the main stairs. I descended into the depths and emerged into a bright corridor with—at last—a sign indicating that the radiotherapy department was around the corner.

I checked in with the receptionist and sat down in the small waiting room. A Chinese woman was sitting with an older lady, maybe her mother? The younger had a pretty headscarf covering her (I presumed, hairless) head. She stared into space, hunched forward. In the corner of the room a man lay motionless on a trolley. A nurse was fiddling with his various monitors. An elderly couple sat opposite me, both wrapped in scarves and coats. He carried a stick, her knuckles were white as she gripped her small handbag to her stomach. I wondered which one of them was the patient. I seemed very healthy in contrast, other than my infected wound I felt OK.

'Kathleen Thompson?' The elderly nurse's query interrupted my thoughts.

'Yes?'

'Would you like to come through?' she led me into a small office,

'This is Dr Peters.' She gestured at the tall man sitting by the desk, before closing the door as she left.

'Hello, do sit down.' His arm stretched towards the vacant chair.

Relaxed and languid, right ankle resting on left thigh, he turned the pages of my notes with long fingers, 'I see Mrs Grant removed the tumour completely. That's good. So the next step is three weeks of radiotherapy to your right breast, followed by a week's 'boost' to the area of the tumour bed. OK?' he reached for the consent form on his desk as he spoke.

'Yes. I do have a few questions.'

'Oh? Oh, OK, yes, well fire away.' His hand hovered in the air, holding the consent form, which was a booklet several pages thick.

'Well, I've been told that the radiotherapy can cause fibrosis in the breast, and it may cause it to shrink and become small and hard?'

'Not in my unit.' He fixed my eyes and smiled as he pulled the consent form back towards him. He started filling in my name and hospital details, 'Women with very large breasts do sometimes get fibrosis, but you should be fine.'

He swung back slightly on his chair, 'Anything else?'

'I'm taking tamoxifen at the moment – should I stop it whilst I'm having the radiotherapy?'

'No, it should be fine. Just carry on with it.'

'Are there any vitamins or supplements which would help? Or any that I shouldn't take during the treatment?'

'You shouldn't really need supplements with a normal healthy diet. But you can take them if you like. It shouldn't be a problem.'

He started to tick some of the boxes on the consent form. He looked up and paused,

'Well, if you don't have any more questions, I just need you to sign this.' He leant across the desk and placed the booklet in front of me, open on the signature page, 'There, just sign there and date it.'

I knew I should read it before signing it, but I felt embarrassed. He'd only offered me the signature page, and he was holding the pen out for me to sign. How could I insist on reading the whole form without appearing to doubt his integrity? After all, I wasn't buying a car from a dodgy salesman, was I? I tried to quickly scan the only page visible and noticed that he'd ticked the box stating that breast fibrosis was a potential side-effect, which seemed odd after his reassurance that it shouldn't be a problem. I also noticed that he hadn't ticked the box marked 'Tiredness.'

'I see you didn't tick 'Tiredness', but lots of people have told me I will feel tired, isn't that the case?'

'No, not really.' he smiled at me, but I noticed his gaze slipped down to the signature line. I must be holding him up. I didn't have the guts to challenge him again about the breast fibrosis. I signed.

He took the signed form and put it in my notes. He didn't give me a copy to read.

'OK, so we'll book you in for the planning CAT scan today. Basically we use the CAT scan to plan exactly how much radiotherapy to give you, and exactly what direction the beams should go. We'll take lots of measurements, and we'll put some small tattoos on your skin. That way, when you start the radiotherapy, we can line you up each time in exactly the same position and make sure that we are always treating exactly the right place.

'When you have the planning scan, we'll give you your appointment times for the four weeks of treatment. That way you can organise your life.' his smile was genuinely sympathetic now.

'Well thank you, Dr Peters.' I got up and left the room. He closed the door behind me immediately.

I sat back in the waiting room and waited for the nurse to bring my appointment. I didn't know what to think. He'd seemed competent and friendly, and he'd said what I wanted to hear, that my breast wouldn't become shrunken and hard after the radiotherapy. I was only too willing to believe him. His didactic responses hadn't really encouraged further discussion. I was nervous of the radiotherapy, and I wanted to believe it would all go well.

The nurse walked over to me, carrying a small white card, 'This is your planning appointment. Come about 15 minutes early if you can, so we can fill in our questionnaires and go through the process with you.'

'Yes, OK. Thank you.'

We're required to sign a consent form for major treatments, such as surgery or radiotherapy. Doctors vary in their attitude towards this. I described Mrs

Grant's consent procedure earlier, which was an excellent example of how to make sure the patient really does understand the procedure before agreeing to it.

In contrast, Dr Peters appeared to regard the form primarily as an administrative procedure. He was not unusual in that respect—in fact I would say that Mrs. Grant's approach is probably less common. I don't mean to imply that Dr Peters was trying to persuade me to accept treatment against my better judgement. Of course not, I am certain that his intentions were sincere, and many patients really just want to sign the form and have done with it too. Nevertheless the informed consent procedure is an important opportunity to make sure the patient is making the best decision for their needs and circumstances, which may not always be the recommended choice of the medical profession.

You should at least have a chance to read the consent form thoroughly and to ask questions without feeling pressured. You should also be given your own copy to take away.

You do need to consider how you ask questions too. If I'm honest, my enquiry about fibrosis was worded towards getting the answer I wanted. I could have simply asked whether any fibrosis would develop. But I didn't, I exaggerated, I asked if my breast would become shrunken and hard. Dr Peters responded to that particular question and confirmed that it wouldn't, but omitted to add that it didn't mean I wouldn't get any fibrosis at all.

We were both subconsciously colluding. I had geared my question to get the negative response I wanted, and he obliged. If you really want to know the truth, you have to phrase your question honestly.

Dr Peters seemed preoccupied and busy. He probably was—his department treated many very serious cancers. My case was comparatively simple and straightforward, and I was actually very lucky.

However to me, my cancer was both serious and important. If I sensed that Dr Peters was busy and didn't have a lot of time to spend on a relatively straightforward case like mine, I should have ignored it. The consultation was my time, and if I needed him to give me time to go through my worries I should have demanded it. I should have quizzed him about ticking fibrosis on the consent form, I should have asked him to take me through the consent form. I should have sat glued to that wooden chair in his office until I was satisfied.

In all honesty I'm sure Dr Peters would have been horrified to know that I'd left feeling confused and unhappy. People are often busy in hospitals, but most of them genuinely want to do a good job for their patients and will give you time if they know you need it.

The next step before my radiotherapy was the planning CAT scan. This would involve lying under another large metal machine – called a simulator, because it simulates your radiotherapy treatment. You have to lie in the same position as for your radiotherapy—usually on your back, with the arm on the treatment side above your head. Small metal markers, which show up on X-rays, will be sellotaped around your breasts to help orientate the doctor who is planning the treatment. Various X-ray images will be taken.

A CAT scan is a series of X-ray images taken from many different angles and then merged by computer to produce a picture which looks as if someone has taken a slice right through you (the old 'saw the lady in half' magicians' trick, but without the pain or blood).

After the CAT scan, permanent dark blue marks are tattooed on your chest at the site of the metal markers. This allows the radiographers who will give the radiotherapy to make sure that for each treatment you are in exactly the same position as you were at the planning session, so that the radiation is aimed at the correct place each time.

My Story

Two weeks later I was in the department again, waiting for my planning CAT scan. I'd popped in to see Bronwen on the way.

She was pleased with my wound, 'Slowly closing up, Kathleen. Book in to see me in about a week, when you're coming for your radiotherapy.'

I left Bronwen and walked down the narrow steps to the radiotherapy department—slowly. I was in no hurry. I was worrying about the tattoos. I'd coped with the surgery. I'd been quite upbeat. Mrs Grant had done a great job and I was happy with my new body. But now I was going to have permanent, dark blue marks in my cleavage, and just above my breast. After all I'd been through, all the efforts to restore my femininity, to make my body look normal, they were going to disfigure me with these blue marks. There'd be a third mark too, but it would be hidden under my arm, so I was less concerned about that one.

I sat in the small waiting room, hugging my knees. I ignored the pile of dated magazines and stared around the room. I tried to remind myself that I was lucky. Many others waiting had much more serious problems. My treatment was just preventative. I'd an excellent chance of kicking the cancer for good. But it didn't help, the small tattoos had grown to the size of huge inky blots in my mind.

A door opened, and a tall dark-haired man came out and smiled at me, 'Kathleen Thompson?'

'Yes'

'Hi. I'm Christopher, one of the radiotherapy assistants. Could you come with me please?'

I followed him back into the small room.

'So, today's your planning session.'

He went on to explain the procedure, but I could hardly concentrate. Eventually he asked if I had any questions.

'How big exactly will the tattoos be?' I blurted out.

He grinned, 'Everyone worries about the tattoos. They'll be the size of this freckle,' he pointed to his wrist, 'about 2mm across – really tiny. They'll look like a blackhead.' his voice faded with his last comment. Maybe it occurred to him that having permanent 'blackheads' displayed every time I wore a low-cut dress may not be the best selling point.

'Don't worry, they're really small.' he repeated quietly.

'Oh, just one last thing, are you happy to allow trainee staff to be involved with your care?'

'Yes, that's fine.'

'OK. You don't have to agree, but if you're sure, I'll make a note.'

'No, it's fine.' I didn't see a problem. People had to learn, and any trainees would be supervised. I remembered learning that way myself as a medical student many years earlier.

'Lovely. Well that's it. Just pop outside and someone will call you in for the scan.'

A few minutes later, a young radiographer sauntered into the waiting room where I was sitting, carrying a set of notes, 'Agnes Thompson?' she called out.

Nobody answered. I was puzzled. My second name was Agnes. Did she mean me? I asked her.

'Oh yes, Kathleen Agnes Thompson' she replied flatly. I read her name badge: 'Esme Smith, trainee radiographer'.

I followed her into the CAT scan suite. Three radiographers were walking around the large machine which dominated the room, checking various dials. As per usual, I was asked to strip to the waist and wear a blue gown.

The radiographer who seemed to be in charge was a middle-aged man with gold-rimmed glasses and black hair.

'Hello, my name's Michael. Please lie down here under the simulator and undo your gown.'

His manner was polite but cold. Although I'd stripped to the waist in front of strangers on a regular basis since my diagnosis, I felt oddly vulnerable and embarrassed lying there semi-naked in front of him. He leant over me and made some marks with a black felt-tip pen on my skin, then stuck some strips of metal around the perimeter of my breasts. He explained that these strips would be visible on the CAT scan, and the markings were where the tattoos would be placed.

As he did this, the other two radiographers continued to look at the machine controls and make notes. Esme, the trainee radiographer stood motionless by the door, staring, her mouth slightly open.

After a lot of activity Michael eventually said, 'Right, please lie very still. We'll take some X-rays now.' They all left the room.

I lay there motionless, as requested. After less than a minute they came back in, and Michael strode over to where I was lying.

He leant towards me. I noticed Esme was standing to his left.

He pushed her forward. 'Esme's going to place your tattoos now.'

As her face floated above me, she had the same vacant expression as when she'd misread my name. I shrank into the trolley.

Surely SHE wasn't going to do the tattoos? Did she know what she was doing? Yes, I'd agreed trainees could be involved in my care, but I hadn't really expected someone to practice on me with the tattoos. All my fears about them over the last two weeks bubbled up and steamed around my head.

What could I do? If I said that I didn't want her to do them, I'd appear unreasonable, and anyway I had no reason to tell them that she'd do badly. I remembered Christopher had assured me that I didn't have to agree to students—I could object. But I was caught off guard. My mind went blank. I couldn't think of any acceptable objection, so I said nothing.

Michael's gold-rimmed spectacles glinted under the large lights, as the girl, with shaking hands and expressionless face, stabbed at my chest with a sharp instrument, like a small pen, coated in dark blue ink. First in my cleavage, then above my right breast, then finally under my right arm. She was slow and awkward, making a couple of attempts with the first two. She seemed to dig really hard and deep. She struggled to reach the last one though, right under my arm, and didn't spend long on it. Just one quick stab.

She stepped back when she'd finished.

'Well done Esme' Michael murmured.

I looked down at my chest. The two tattoos on my front looked much larger than freckles. I estimated that one was almost half a centimeter across. Then I looked under my right arm – the third tattoo was small and faint – hardly visible, but that wouldn't have mattered anyway as it was hidden. I felt violated. I didn't think she'd done well. In fact I strongly suspected she'd never done it before.

I just wanted them to finish and let me out of there. I lay frozen, unable to think, just doing whatever they asked me until finally I was able to go. I rushed to the nearest Ladies, locked myself in the cubicle and pulled up my jumper and stared in the small mirror. It looked a mess - all that expert surgery, the carefully hidden scars, and now these ugly black marks. I snatched a crumpled tissue and wiped away the tears. I took a few deep breaths and tried to steel myself to face the world, to get myself home.

My reaction may seem a little over the top. After all, two small blue-black marks on my skin were hardly devastating in the grand scheme of preventing me dying from cancer. Somehow it mattered a lot to me, though. My emotions were still overactive—my whole life had been turned upside down, my frames of reference were no longer reliable. It just seemed another assault on my body image, on top of everything else.

Maybe I'd have felt reassured if the tattoos really had been the small freckles I'd been promised. It was unfortunate that mine were done by a trainee and that she had made the two visible ones bigger than I'd been led to expect. It was also unfortunate that once again, I hadn't voiced my concerns. I could have been pleasant and assertive—pointing out that I was worried about the tattoos and would feel more confident with someone experienced doing them.

Why the hell hadn't I spoken up? Partly I was taken by surprise. Michael had told me as a *fait accompli*, and psychologically I was at a disadvantage—

lying beneath them semi-naked. Trainees have to learn, and most of the time they are well supervised and do a good job. But even if you have agreed that they can be involved with your care—and that is entirely up to you—you can still change your mind if you're not happy.

Medical staff should also be aware that 'consent' isn't freely given if the patient hasn't had a fair chance to consider and refuse. Michael should have sat me up and asked if I minded if Esme did the tattoos, offering me the alternative of an experienced member of staff. Then at least I would have had a fair opportunity to say no. Having said that, patients weren't always given much chance to refuse my inexpert administrations when I was training either. Maybe this was some weird karma coming back to bite me, but it still wasn't right.

My concern about the tattoos was that they were permanent and ugly, plus they would forever stigmatize me as an ex-cancer sufferer. I was told that the tattoos needed to be permanent in case I ever needed radiotherapy again, at which point it would be necessary to know exactly which parts of my body had received how much radiation, as there is a maximum safe dose which can be given to any one place.

At the end of my treatment, I asked Dr Peters if I could undergo laser treatment to remove the tattoos. He said yes, because I was a low risk patient and because they'd also taken photographs which could be used to work out where the tattoos had been, if ever needed.

If this was the case, why had I been given permanent tattoos?

I suspect a more compelling argument was that it was to make absolutely sure that the tattoos didn't disappear during the current course of treatment, rather than any concern over future therapy. Radiotherapy can last many weeks and the radiographers need the tattoos to line you up precisely each time.

However, as you will see in the subsequent chapter, steps can be taken if the tattoos do fade, and staff can go over them with biros to make sure they stay visible. If your cancer is more serious, and there is a significant risk that you will need further radiotherapy, then it may be important to have permanent tattoos. But if this is not the case, semi-permanent tattoos exist, and if you find the idea of permanent tattoos upsetting, you could ask about these.

After your treatment is finished, if you want to remove permanent tattoos, you should discuss it with your radiotherapist first in case there is an important reason why you shouldn't. Laser treatment removes most tattoos. It isn't available on the NHS, but there are many places that provide this service. I would advise you to check the qualifications of the operator—lasers can cause damage and scarring if used incorrectly. I telephoned a few, and frankly there were some that I wouldn't have trusted to laser my dustbin.

I eventually found a practice run by a doctor and a nurse. I spoke to the nurse and felt confident in her abilities. Unfortunately, it turned out that Esme had done a very thorough job, and, although the marks faded slightly, they never fully disappeared. I have gradually become less sensitive about them, and I use concealer to hide them if necessary. However, people do occasionally comment on them, and it was a whole load of emotional anguish I could have managed without.

Summary:

Radiotherapy damages cancer cells more than healthy ones
It can be used to treat breast cancer, but it is also used after surgery to prevent the cancer coming back
Currently, a typical regime would last 4 weeks in total
A single treatment given during the breast operation is being investigated
During treatment your skin will probably become sore and red
You may suffer breast swelling, or shrinking, and thickening, which may be long-term.
Other rare effects may occur
A radiotherapist is a doctor specializing in this area
Cancer statistics can be confusing. Make sure you understand exactly what they mean for you
Before your radiotherapy starts your treatment will be carefully planned, using CAT scanning.
Tattoos are needed to make sure your treatment is directed accurately
Semi-permanent tattoos are sometimes adequate
You can have laser treatment to remove or fade tattoos
You can and should object if worried about a trainee performing a procedure

Further Information:

Planning (Cancer Research UK)	http://goo.gl/I8nF1j
BreastCancer.org	http://goo.gl/EnPbzL
About (Cancer Research UK)	http://goo.gl/ncWrn8
Side Effects (Cancer Research UK)	http://goo.gl/xhY018
Breast Cancer Care	https://goo.gl/jEn9Ls

Chapter 21

Radiotherapy—getting through the treatment

My Story

After the planning, it was nearly two weeks before my first radiotherapy treatment. My appointments schedule for the full four weeks was filed in the large, untidy 'to do' pile on my desk.

I was monitoring the tattoos every day. The two on my front were large and blue-black as ever but the one under my arm, which had started off tiny, had been gradually but definitely fading. By the Friday before my treatment started on the Monday, I could hardly see it at all. I knew they needed all three tattoos, to line me up accurately. Would there be anything at all to see by the first session?

I hardly slept that whole weekend. By Monday morning I couldn't see the third tattoo at all. I had a direct number for my radiotherapy key worker, Sunita. I waited until 9am, then phoned. The number rang and rang. Eventually the general switchboard told me I'd been given an incorrect number. They put me through to Sunita.

I hadn't met her, but I poured out my worries to her. She was calm and sympathetic. 'Don't worry,' she said. 'I'm sure we'll be able to see the tattoo, even if it's very small. We took photographs too, so we can use skin marks like moles to help find it.'

'But what if you can't?'

'Well if we really can't, we'd have to re-do the CAT scan, but you mustn't worry, just come along this afternoon and I'll see you then.'

I was unable to concentrate on anything as I walked to the hospital. It was about three miles from the station, but walking calmed me down, and the weather was warm and pleasant.

I trailed down the narrow staircase and presented myself to the young Chinese receptionist. He always seemed to be smiling.

'Hi there. Just walk down the corridor to the radiotherapy suite. I'll call Sunita.'

I did as he asked and found a vacant seat against the wall. There was nobody else around.

A few minutes later, a door marked 'Do Not Enter' opened, and a young Indian girl emerged and sat next to me, 'Hi, I'm Sunita,' she said.

Her long shiny pony-tail hung down her back as she checked her paperwork.

'OK, first I need you to tell me your full name and date of birth.' She looked up, 'You'll get really fed up of us asking you this, but it's part of our procedure. We have to make sure we're giving the right patient the right treatment.'

'That's perfect. Right, let me explain. I'm going to take you into the room with the radiotherapy machine in a few minutes. You'll need to put on a blue gown then lie under the machine, a bit like when you had the planning CAT-scan. The radiographers will move you about on the couch until your tattoos line up with the machine, then they'll all leave the room while we give you the treatment. You need to lie very still at that point, but don't worry, they'll be watching you all the time, and if you need to attract their attention just raise your left arm. Did you put deodorant on today?'

'Yes I did. I didn't think the radiotherapy would go into my armpit. The lymph nodes were clear'.

'Oh, you shouldn't use deodorant. It contains metals which can make your skin burn. Don't worry I'll wipe it off when you're in the room.'

'OK, but what about my tattoo. You remember I phoned you? The one under my arm has disappeared.'

'I'm sure the radiographers'll find it, don't worry. Just wait there a few more minutes and I'll be back.' She smiled and left.

Five minutes later another radiographer took me into the treatment room. I looked around. It was a big, well-lit space with a large radiotherapy machine in the middle and a couch underneath. There was no sign of Sunita.

I was given the familiar blue gown and ushered towards a small alcove in a corner of the room. A curtain was suspended from a square-shaped rail on the ceiling. It could be pulled round, for privacy. But I knew I would soon be told to open the blue gown and display myself to everyone in the room, so I didn't bother.

A male radiographer asked me to lie on the couch under the machine, then open my gown. Once again I felt embarrassed without knowing quite why. Maybe it was because it only seemed OK to strip in front of men who were doctors, or maybe I was just generally getting over-sensitive, but everything about the radiotherapy made me feel edgy.

'Can you tell me your name, address and date of birth?' He asked. I told him.

'Now I'm going to move your body slightly to line your tattoos up with our machine. Don't try to help me, just let me move you.'

'But one of the tattoos has disappeared—the one under my arm.'

'Let's take a look.' He studied my side for ages, comparing it with the photographs in the notes he was holding.

'It's OK. It is extremely faint but I can just about make it out.' As he spoke he drew a large cross over the faded tattoo with a biro.

Relief washed over me like a warm shower. Thank God. I made a mental note to avoid washing his biro mark.

I allowed him to shift my body until my tattoos lined up with the black cross targets projected from the radiotherapy machine onto my skin.

All the while he was engaged in a running dialogue with his colleague. Each of them was carefully checking measurements, and they confirmed every single measurement with each other, to make sure that the radiotherapy exposure was exactly as planned. This procedure was followed before every one of my treatments. The radiographers who specialized in radiotherapy were all very competent and careful. Dr Peters seemed to run a tight ship.

'OK, lie very still. We'll take an X-ray before this first dose, and then we'll give you the treatment straight afterwards.'

They left the room.

I felt nervous as I lay there. The twenty sessions I needed seem to stretch out for ever. I thought of my mother. She'd needed radiotherapy for her breast cancer just one year earlier. She'd been terrified too, and I'd been so unfeeling. I remembered thinking that all she had to do was lie there for a few minutes while some X-rays were beamed at her. How hard was that?

Well now I understood just how hard it was. I'd regarded the radiotherapy beam as healing rays in my mother's case, magically dissolving her large tumour. Now they'd taken on a completely different identity. They were destructive rays, searing through my body, frying my tissues as they went, causing lasting shrinkage and fibrosis. My imagination was expanding faster than a mushroom cloud.

Then, as I lay there, I suddenly remembered that Sunita had promised to wipe *away my deodorant so my skin wouldn't burn.*

The large machine was circumscribing an arc through the air above me, and I wasn't sure whether it was still taking X-rays or whether they'd started the radiotherapy. Remembering Sunita's instructions I kept still, but raised my left arm to attract their attention. Meanwhile the radiation machine had reached my right side. It was directed inwards and upwards towards my right breast. No one responded to my waving hand, and it occurred to me that if the radiotherapy had started, my left hand and arm would have been in direct line of fire. Oh great, I thought.

A few minutes later the radiographers came back into the room. One told me I could get dressed and go. I mentioned about the deodorant but he didn't seem interested.

As I walked back to the train station I felt quite numb. It was a strange, almost anticlimactic feeling. I'd feared the radiotherapy so much, but it hadn't actually hurt—in fact it hadn't appeared to have had any effect at all.

Another nineteen doses left. Well, I felt OK so far, but I was longing for it all to be over.

By the fourth treatment I'd started to relax. Nothing terrible had happened, and I was starting to get to know some of the staff. The young Chinese receptionist greeted me by name now.

Every day, even the staff who knew me asked me my name, date of birth and address before they gave me the treatment. There were lots of radiographers in the department. I felt an instant empathy with some—but not all.

I had been assigned to a particular radiotherapy machine. They all had strange and unmemorable names, which I suspected acknowledged generous benefactors.

Halfway through the second week, 'my' machine was out of action—undergoing maintenance, they told me, so the receptionist directed me to another machine. I instantly forgot the strange name he'd told me and wandered around the department, a little confused, trying to find where I should go.

I bumped into Christopher, the assistant who'd explained things on the planning day.

'Hi, are you OK? You look lost.'

'Yes, my machine's out of action and I'm not sure where I'm supposed to go.'

'What's the name of the machine you need?'

'What?' I replied 'Listen, you normally ask me easy questions like my name and date of birth. Now you're asking me the machine's name?'

'Yes, and my next question was, what's the square root of 956?' he winked.

'Hang on here, I'll find out where you're supposed to be.'

When he returned, he took me to a different waiting area, which I noticed was slightly more comfortable than my usual spot. It was empty, so I sat on the small sofa and waited.

I heard a noise and looked up. A middle-aged gentleman was standing at the entrance. He oozed self-importance, and his impeccable grey suit was definitely more Savile Row than M&S. He surveyed the room, giving me a cursory, dismissive look, and sat down, as far away from me as possible, as if he thought low social status may be contagious.

Just then a radiographer came out and asked me in a clear voice whether I was Dr Thompson. She then checked a couple of details with me and left again.

Ha! I thought, rather childishly, that'll show him.

Immediately the radiographer returned and, addressing the snooty man, smiled and said, 'Would you like to follow me, Sir Christopher?'

I smiled too, to myself. He'd trumped my title fair and square.

By the end of the second week, I was beginning to feel the effects of the radiation. I felt OK until I tried to do anything, then I'd feel tired and achy, as if I had a bug. I wondered if my symptoms were also partly due to my many sleepless nights. My anxiety levels were still running high. I was also trying to keep up my yoga and pilates classes, and I was walking to the hospital from the station, around three miles each way. I didn't always manage it, sometimes I took the bus, but I pushed myself as much as I could. Maybe this was why I felt so tired? I didn't do 'taking it easy' very well.

It's strange. It was almost as if I gave off an aura of vulnerability, because I experienced several examples of kindness from total strangers over that time. On one occasion it was raining hard and I was feeling exhausted. A bus was stopping at a crowded bus stop. I saw a man get on and then off again, and return to the queue. Without thinking, I dragged myself onto the platform. There was no room to move. The driver shouted at me, 'Move down, you can't stand in the entrance.'

I pushed further along, and as I did so a young woman offered me her seat. It wasn't until later that I realised that the driver had been turning people off the full bus, yet he'd let me get on. Somehow he and the young woman seemed to sense my need.

On another occasion, an elderly Indian man stood patiently holding the door for me for ages, while I walked the length of a corridor.

On a different day, I stood back to let a pretty young black woman pass with a pushchair. I suppose I was staring. Actually I was wondering what awful reason had brought her and her child into a cancer hospital? As she passed me, she flashed me a shy smile and whispered, 'I love your skirt.'

Little kindnesses meant a lot, and I seemed to be getting more than my fair share.

Meanwhile I was still seeing Bronwen every week. She seemed to have a large variety of wound dressings in her repertoire, to cope with the various stages of healing. When the alginate dressing failed to mop up all the gunge, she changed it for a more absorbent dressing. As the wound began to dry up, she produced another, which looked like felt, and which drew the edges of the wound together.

At this stage I started to struggle with my diet. I craved carbohydrates and sweet things because I was so tired. I knew I shouldn't—there's a direct link between being overweight and breast cancer—and I knew my best chance of disease-free survival was to control my natural tendency to put on weight. I even made posters for my kitchen cupboard to remind me to be good, but it was amazing how rapidly I developed selective blindness as I reached for the biscuit tin.

My skin was starting to get red and sore too. Bronwen had been right, it felt just like sunburn. It peeled slightly, and I had to be careful not to rub it too hard, as it was quite delicate. It wasn't too troublesome though. I took her advice and used aloe vera on it (when I remembered).

Overall, the radiotherapy wasn't as bad as I'd feared. If I hadn't had preconceptions about it, maybe it would have been even easier. But I'm human, and we can't always be perfectly rational all the time. You may react negatively to some or all aspects of your treatment. Just because someone else found it easy doesn't mean you are being a wimp.

Please be easy on yourself—you are going through a lot, physically and emotionally.

Summary:

At first you probably won't feel any effect of the radiotherapy
After a week or so your skin will appear sunburned
Aloe vera can help
You may start to feel tired – partly due to the treatment, but maybe due to other reasons too, such as stress

Further Information:

See previous chapter.

Chapter 22

Radiotherapy boost—challenging medical decisions

My Story

During my second week of radiotherapy I was given an appointment with Dr Peters to plan my final week of treatment—the 'boost'. This is where the immediate area that had surrounded my tumour would be zapped. Since Phil had moved house I hadn't seen so much of him, but he came to stay for a few days, and came to the appointment with me. He knew it was important.

I had my radiotherapy first, then Fern, one of the radiographers, took us to the outpatient department. The three of us waited in the consulting room for Dr Peters.

A tall, slim young doctor popped his head around the door. 'Sorry to keep you, I'll be with you in a minute.' he smiled, and left.

'Who's he, Fern?' I asked the radiographer, 'I thought I was seeing Dr Peters?'

'Oh, he's one of the registrars.'

The doctor returned and sat down.

'Hello, I'm Dr. Ernest.' he stared at me through dark-rimmed glasses, blond wavy hair framing his pale face. 'I see you're a doctor yourself—what sort of doctor?' he asked.

'I'm a paediatrician, but now I work in the pharmaceutical industry.' I replied.

'I see. Well today I'm going to plan your radiotherapy boost. 'Your X-rays show the tumour was in your right breast, around two o'clock, is that correct?' (He was using the clock-face to describe where in my breast the tumour had been).

'No, it was lower than that—three o'clock.' I replied.

'Really?' he looked puzzled. 'I'll go and check the mammogram again, but I'm

173

confident it was two o'clock.'

He left the room for a few minutes, 'Yep, definitely two o'clock.' he announced as he walked back through the door.

I was sure he was wrong, but I couldn't think what to say without accusing him of being incompetent, or a liar, or both. So I kept quiet, but my mind was racing.

'OK, could you take your top things off and lie down here. I'm going to draw a circle on your breast where you'll have your boost, then Fern here will make a template and take some photographs.'

As I lay on the couch, he leaned over me and laid a Perspex sheet on my breast. The sheet had circular holes cut out of it of varying sizes. It reminded me of a child's stencil set.

He chose a largish hole and with a black felt tip pen he drew a circle on my breast around the edge of the hole. 'This is more of an art than a science,' he said.

I could barely concentrate, as he continued drawing an innocent-looking black felt-tip circle—in what I was absolutely sure was the wrong place. I tried once more to protest that I was sure the area was wrong, as the mammogram hadn't shown all the tumour.

He smiled, 'Look, don't worry. I'm using quite a large circle, so even if it was at three o'clock, this circle will cover that area too.'

Surely the idea of the boost was to treat only the area where the tumour had been, and to avoid damaging the normal breast tissue around it? If he was drawing such a big circle, wasn't he defeating the entire purpose of the treatment? But I didn't argue any more. He was convinced he was right.

I dressed and left with Phil, who spoke as soon as we got outside, 'I remember, it was where you said – I'm sure it was.' He looked worried, and as perplexed and helpless as I felt.

'Let's go home and I'll go through all the letters from the hospital and remind myself. We've still got time to persuade him.' I'd chosen to receive copies of all hospital letters sent to my GP, an option which had been offered to me at my first appointment at the Breast Unit. As soon as I got home I dug out the letters.

There it was, clearly written, 'tumour at 3 o'clock'. I started to relax. I was right and I could prove it. I made copies of all the relevant letters, highlighting the statements about the tumour location, and packed them to take to the hospital the following day.

As soon as I got to the radiotherapy department, I found Fern. 'Hello Fern, I wanted to have a chat about my boost treatment.'

'Yes sure, fire away.'

I looked around the crowded waiting room. 'Is there somewhere we can talk privately?'

'Yes, of course, let's go in this office.' She led me into a small but comfortable room.

'Fern, I checked my hospital letters when I got home. Dr Ernest used my mammogram to place my tumour, but I had lots more tests. The MRI scan showed it was actually lower down - the mammogram had only shown part of it. Here, you see?' I pointed to the highlighted sections on the letters I was clutching.

'OK. Can I take these to my supervisor?'

'Yes, these are your copies. I've highlighted the key information.'

'Thanks, that's perfect.'

She went away, returning after a few minutes. 'We've had a chat. We'll discuss this at the multidisciplinary team meeting, and I've made you an appointment to see Dr Peters next Monday. Your boost isn't until another week after that, so we've plenty of time.'

I heaved a sigh of relief. Mrs Grant would be at the team meeting. She'd confirm that the tumour had been lower down. Dr Peters would move the area of the boost dose and everything would be fine.

By the Friday of that week I was feeling low and weepy. The skin over the radiotherapy area had become quite red and sore now. As the redness developed, I could see exactly where the radiation had hit my body. The area seemed to include a lot more normal tissue than I was expecting, including my armpit. If the lymph nodes there were damaged I was at risk of lymphoedema (permanent swelling) in my arm. I was also concerned that my back muscle seemed to have been caught in the radiation field too, as it passed over the back of my armpit. I asked a radiographer if this was OK.

'Mention it to Dr Peters on Monday,' he replied.

My right hand had also started to develop pins and needles. Had the radiotherapy caused damage to the nerves to my hand as they passed through my armpit? Or was it the blood vessels which had been affected?

I could be left with a permanent swelling of my arm, or numbness, or maybe it would become partially paralysed. My head was spinning with all these fears, some rational, some exaggerated—with no one to really reassure me until Monday. I had the weekend to get through first.

Monday morning came. Phil had come to stay again, God bless him. We set off for my appointment with Dr Peters. I'd made another copy of the relevant hospital letters to take with me, just in case the last set had been mislaid.

We got there early, descended into the depths of the earth and, after a quick greeting from the smiley Receptionist, sat and waited.

Eventually a nurse called us in. As I walked into the room, I saw Dr Peters sitting at the desk, and Dr Ernest leaning against the examination couch.

Dr. Peters greeted us, 'Good morning. Please sit down. So what's the problem here?'

'Good morning Dr Peters, Dr Ernest. Nice to see you both,' I replied, as Phil and I sat down on the small wooden chairs. 'Last week Dr Ernest and I were discussing where my tumour had been. From the mammogram he thought it was at 2 o'clock, but in fact the MRI scan showed up more of the tumour and...'

'We used the MRI to decide where the boost should go.' Dr Peters cut through my explanation.

Startled by his response, I lost my thread. Did he mean they'd looked at my MRI scan together, after my last appointment? Maybe they'd gone through it with Mrs Grant at the multidisciplinary meeting?

'Oh, OK, good,' I replied.

'Yes, we used the MRI scan. The siting is correct.' Dr Peters's lips were tight and pale.

Surely I wasn't hearing right. Surely he wasn't refusing to acknowledge the mistake? Refusing to even discuss the information in the letters I'd given them?

I tried again, but every time I started to talk, Dr Peters talked across me, so I was unable to finish. It was hopeless.

'But I remember,' Phil spoke. 'The needle holes from the biopsies were lower down too...'

'That doesn't mean anything. You can go through the same hole to biopsy different areas. It doesn't mean that's where the tumour was.' Dr Ernest interrupted him.

Dr Peters seemed irritated now. The atmosphere in the small room was crackling.

'Anyway, the boost area I've drawn is large enough to cover where you thought the tumour was.' Dr Ernest continued.

Why did he seem to think accuracy was so unimportant? Phil and I lapsed into silence, staring at Dr Peters. I was feeling hot, my palms were damp. I shifted in my seat. I couldn't breathe, it was too stuffy. I wanted to get out, get some fresh air.

'So, have you any further questions?' Dr Peters asked.

The hard chair pressed painfully against my shoulder blades and back, as I sagged into it. I decided to ask about the other things that had been worrying me. I may as well get something out of the consultation. 'I've been getting some numbness in my right arm for the last few days. Could the radiotherapy be affecting my nerves? From the areas of reddened skin, the radiation seems to be going right into my armpit?'

Dr Peters leaned slowly towards me, 'Well you'd be my first patient if it had.'

He paused, sat back, took a breath then carried on, 'Nerve damage is rare and it doesn't appear for months after treatment, so no, your numbness isn't due to the radiotherapy.'

'OK. Also, I've noticed from the skin marks, that the radiotherapy seems to have gone outside the breast. Could it damage the lymph nodes there?'

'Some lymph nodes do get hit by the radiotherapy anyway. That's probably why patients do well even if the surgeon hasn't done a perfect job.' he gave a wry smile.

I sagged further into my chair, drained.

'Anything else worrying you?' Dr Peters spoke more gently now.

'No, thank you.'

We stumbled out of the room. I felt dazed and hopeless, resigned to the idea that my boost would be directed at the wrong area. Not only that, but I felt embarrassed. Would Dr Peters complain about me to Mrs Grant? Would someone write 'Trouble-maker' in my notes? Would the attitude of other staff members change towards me? What about the people whom I'd grown to respect and admire, such as Bronwen. Would her genuine, caring smile harden next time she saw me?

Phil stayed a couple of days more before going home. Over that time, we talked about what had happened. We both felt impotent. If the consultant himself refused to listen, what could we do? I was grateful for Phil's attempt to defend me, it had got nowhere. It wasn't right. I was a patient. What was wrong with them?

My experience highlights the importance of taking responsibility for your own treatment. Don't just assume other people will do everything correctly. People are human, they don't always get things right, and at the final reckoning you're the person who has most to lose. So if the hospital asks if you would like copies of the letters they send out, say yes. And when they arrive, keep them all together in a small file. You may need to refer to them later. I had changed hospitals, so I anticipated that there might be some communication breakdowns.

But the communication breakdown had taken place within the same hospital. This shouldn't have happened. The whole point of weekly multi-disciplinary team meetings was to avoid exactly this situation. The operation notes would have clearly stated where the tumour had been. However the radiotherapy department seemed to use a completely separate set of notes from the surgeons', as far as I could tell. It appeared to me that Dr Ernest was relying on my mammogram, despite Dr Peters' assertion otherwise.

Even if you are convinced there has been a mistake, as my case illustrates, it isn't always an easy matter to get things changed.

So what happened to me?

My Story

I continued to visit the radiotherapy department for my daily treatments. I still had another week to go before the boost started.

Whenever Bronwen checked my wound, the radiotherapy department would give me their notes to take to her. After my meeting with Drs Peters and Ernest, I felt paranoid. The next time I had my notes, I took a detour to the ladies' loo, where I took photos of every page with my phone. I wanted to check that everything was being done properly. I had lost my trust in Dr Peters.

On the Friday, I got back home from my radiotherapy late in the afternoon. I was weary; my right breast had a bad case of sunburn and the soreness extended under my arm, and to the back of my armpit. My back ached, and I felt low and depressed.

I took off my coat and made myself a cup of tea and, feeling guilty as always, I grabbed the cake I'd bought on the way home. I sank onto the sofa and turned on the TV. Peeling the plastic wrapper off the large cupcake, I opened my mouth and let the sweet icing melt on my tongue, before chewing the soft butterscotch-flavoured sponge. I flicked through the channels. Some mindless game show or other, yet another blasted antiques program, cookery program after cookery program (no wonder we're all getting fat, I thought, taking another bite of the cupcake) and a repeat of a chat-show.

With nothing to distract me, my mind inevitably wandered back to my major worry. I went over the consultation for the hundredth time. Yet again, I got out my phone to look at the images of the notes. I clicked on the photograph of my breast with the 'boost' circle marked on it. I stared at it, tracing the black felt-tip shape with my eyes, lining it up with the landmarks of my chest. The more I stared, the more I knew it was wrong. I measured it every which way. It was clearly not centred on where my tumour had been. I became more and more agitated. The boost started on Monday. They were going to treat the wrong place, and I couldn't make them change it. They'd said it didn't matter, but it did, to me.

I phoned Phil and went over it again with him. 'What can I do? The area's definitely wrong. I've checked again. What can I do? They won't listen. You know they won't listen to me. They're going to treat the wrong area. What's the point of having a boost in the wrong area?'

Finally he managed to interrupt. 'Look, you have to contact the hospital and tell them.'

'But what's the point? You know how we tried to make them listen.'

'You must. Have one more go. If you don't, you'll torture yourself all weekend.'

His firm advice hit home. 'You're right,' I said. 'I'll phone them now, there's still time before they finish for the weekend.'

'OK, let me know how you get on.'

I ended the call, dialled the radiotherapy department and asked for Fern.

'Oh I don't think she's in today.' a young female voice answered. 'Actually none of the radiographers are in here. I'm one of the medical physicists, I'm mending the machine.'

'OK. Could you put me through to the supervisor?' I didn't want to lose time talking to a junior. 5pm Friday was speeding towards me.

'Sure, I'll transfer you.' the pleasant disembodied voice replied. The line went quiet.

A few minutes later, I heard a different woman's voice, 'Hello, I'm sorry, the supervisor isn't here.'

'Well I just need to speak to someone who can help me.' I replied, 'The other lady was a medical physicist, just fixing the machine.'

'Oh yes, OK. Can I help? I'm one of the radiographers.'

'I need to get a message to Dr Peters. I'm having a booster dose on Monday, and I need to talk to him about it. Should I speak to his secretary?'

179

'Yes, you could do that.' She dictated the number, and I called it immediately. His secretary answered straight away, and I asked her if she could pass on my message.

'Oh, Dr Peters isn't around at the moment. Could you speak to him next week?'

'No. That's too late. I need to talk to him about my boost, and the first dose is on Monday. I wonder could I send him an email? I have a few reports I want to bring to his attention.'

'Will it be a very long email?' she sounded doubtful.

I laughed. 'Maybe half a page.'

'Ah OK, it was just when you started talking about reports. Dr Peters is actually away on holiday, but if you email me, I'll send it to his personal email address. Hopefully he'll check it before Monday.'

'That's really helpful. Thanks so much.'

She dictated her email address and I put the phone down and started typing:

> *'Dear Dr Peters*
>
> *Thank you for seeing me on Monday to discuss my booster dose.*
>
> *I felt that I was not able to get my points across then, and I would like to explain my concern once more before dosing starts on Monday, as I am terrified that the siting is incorrect.*
>
> *Dr Ernest based the boost area on the mammogram, but this didn't show the whole tumour. Miss Gomez wrote, 'She has a mass in the medial right breast' and Mrs. Grant stated 'In the right breast medially'. Also, in the radiotherapy planning notes, one of your own medical team wrote 'tumour 3 o'clock'.*
>
> *To be honest I was taken aback when I saw you and no changes were made. Please forgive my persistence, but I am in a state of total anxiety because I don't feel my concerns have been addressed.*
>
> *If you read what I have written, and truly believe that my misgivings are unfounded, I will accept this, but I do need to know that they have been taken seriously.*
>
> *Kind regards*
>
> *Kathleen Thompson'*

Ten minutes after I'd sent the email my phone rang. A new, officious female voice came on the line, 'Hello, this is the senior radiographer speaking. Dr Peters's secretary forwarded your email onto me. I've arranged for you to see Dr Peters in the clinic before your boost on Monday. I'll come along too. We'll discuss your boost then.'

She didn't sound too friendly. I was beginning to feel like Arthur Scargill at a Policeman's Ball, but at least I had one more slim chance of trying to prevent the rapidly approaching mis-siting of my boost.

I phoned Phil and my kids straight away and told them the good news. My daughter, knowing my interest in Japanese, sent me a message saying 'Faito!' with a note explaining that it meant "Fight" in Japanese. Actually the Japanese had just adapted the English word 'Fight', and made it sound Japanese - typical of her wry sense of humour.

Over the weekend I rehearsed what I was going to say to Dr Peters. I had reached saturation point and wanted this sorting.

Monday came and I was standing in the radiotherapy department once again. The smiling Chinese receptionist welcomed me by name and I sat down to wait. Phil had offered to come too, but it would have been another long and tiring drive for him, and I felt it would be less confrontational if I went alone.

Eventually the nurse called me in. I walked in and found Dr Ernest sitting alone.

'I'm sorry, Dr Peters isn't here today.' He looked unsure of my reaction.

'That's fine, I'm very happy to see you.' I replied, and I was. To be frank, I felt I had more chance persuading Dr Ernest than Dr Peters

Dr Ernest took a breath, 'So, explain to me again what your concerns are.'

'Well my tumour was at 3 o'clock, not 2 o'clock. If you give the boost where you're planning, there's the possibility that not all the tumour bed will be treated. I'm also worried that a larger than necessary area of normal breast will be dosed, and as this area will show above my clothing I'd rather not have it damaged unnecessarily.'

'Oh, so you're worried about cosmesis! You didn't mention that before.'

Actually, I was worried about the accuracy of the boost siting – but if he wanted a hook to hang on to, I was happy to let him have one.

'Yes, amongst other things. It may seem vain, but I am concerned about my appearance once all this treatment finishes,' I replied.

He was about to continue, but then he paused, as if he'd just taken in what I'd said. He smiled, and said gently: 'Of course you're not vain.'

I smiled back. We both relaxed a little. He picked up an A4 sheet of hand-

written notes, 'I've been going over all the research on booster therapies over the weekend. Would you like me to take you through it?' He looked straight at me. His defensive stance had melted and he seemed genuinely keen to talk things through.

'Yes, I'd really value that.'

He started to summarize the benefits of radiotherapy boosts to me. Apparently it reduced the risk of local tumour recurrence, but not necessarily overall survival. The benefits were greatest for younger women. For me the overall risk of my tumour recurring would be reduced from 7% to 3%. He went on to explain that some specialists wouldn't recommend me to have a boost at all, as the benefit was quite small.

I listened avidly. At last I felt I was able to make an informed decision, based on facts. After some deliberation, I decided that for me, the difference between 3% and 7% was worth the additional radiation to my body.

'I went to see Dr Bronski this morning,' he went on, 'she's a world expert on tumour X-rays. I showed her your images, and she felt, based on those, that the tumour bed was at three o'clock.' He spoke in an even voice.

He didn't acknowledge that Dr Bronski's opinion supported my argument, and I didn't gloat. I appreciated the time he'd clearly spent, albeit belatedly, trying to find the truth. I also appreciated his honesty.

'Thank you for doing all this research. It really helps me to have all this explained.'

His eyes met mine. 'The reason I get out of bed in a morning and do this job is to try to help people.'

I didn't mind this retort. I truly believed he was sincere. He appeared to have made an error, possibly because all the information may not have been readily available to him—and this was a fault of the system. But I think the real mistake had happened when he and Dr Peters had brushed aside my concerns.

'So,' he continued, 'you've three choices really. Either you decide not to have the boost at all, or you go ahead with it as planned ... or I suppose I could move it a little lower.' He finished quietly.

I forced myself to pause before answering. I was nearly there—so close, but not yet in the bag. 'I'd like you to move the booster site, please.' My emotions were screaming and my heart was thudding, but I kept my voice nonchalant and my face impassive. In my mind, I was coaxing a nervy colt. I had hold of the lead-rein, but any false move and he may startle, break away from me, and gallop off, forever out of reach.

He stiffened. 'OK, I'll get a radiographer to come and help me.'

He left the room and returned a few minutes later with a radiographer. 'Come and lie on the couch and we'll have a look at the boost area.'

I walked over to the couch, removed my jumper and bra and lay down.

'You see, the area I already drew really is in the medial quadrant.' He tried one last time.

I pointed to the centre of the circle, 'Not really, this is the centre. That's definitely above the midline.'

'OK I'll move it downwards a little.'

He traced a new felt-tip circle then said goodbye, wished me well and left.

The radiographer finished preparing the template. She lay a sheet of clear Perspex onto my chest and carefully traced the circle Dr Ernest had drawn onto it. Then she traced the radiotherapy tattoos and the edge of my nipple, so that the Perspex could be positioned accurately on my breast before every treatment, and the boost area accurately marked up and irradiated. When she'd finished, she put the Perspex template in my notes and gave them to me, then sent me straight down to the radiotherapy department for the first dose of my boost treatment.

I don't imagine for one moment that Dr Ernest wanted to dose the wrong area, and I'm certainly not accusing him of not caring. As he'd told me, he did his job because he wanted to help patients with cancer. I was truly relieved that he'd agreed to change the siting. The most important thing for me had been to persist in getting my concerns addressed.

I have gone over what happened many times since. I wondered afterwards whether the confusion related to part of my tumour being cancer and part being DCIS (pre-cancer). I don't really know, it was never adequately discussed. I do believe that, until I wrote the email to Dr Peters, they genuinely hadn't understand my concerns, even though I felt I had explained them clearly.

I had made them reconsider, but it hadn't been easy. My email had been the turning point. I was told later that putting a concern in writing carries more weight than just voicing it.

Most medical staff want to help people and really do have your best interests at heart. And sometimes they are right in their decision and you are wrong. It's important to be open to this possibility. However, personality clashes and misunderstandings can occasionally occur. Some patients are difficult, and some hospital staff are difficult. Each side has its own perspective. But the end of the day, it's your health that's important, and the best way to protect it is to have a good relationship with your medical carers. However, if collaborative discussion has failed, what do you do?

If a junior doctor (any doctor below consultant level, even if very experienced, is called a junior doctor) made the disputed decision, then you should first ask to see the consultant and discuss it with them—in my case I was given an appointment with Dr Peters, the consultant, even without my having specifically requested it, which was good practise.

If you get no resolution with the consultant, though, where do you go? Well, it's worth summarizing the issue in a letter or email to the consultant, as I did.

If the consultant doesn't respond positively, write to the Chief Executive Officer of the hospital. The CEO will usually be concerned enough to intervene, as it is their overall responsibility.

Alternatively—or in addition—you can go back to your GP and ask to be referred to a different consultant for a second opinion.

These are all options, but of course it's difficult to fight when you're unwell. As I mentioned before, it's also difficult to argue with the person responsible for your health. If you need urgent treatment you may not have the luxury of time to write and wait for a response from a hospital CEO either. It's easy to feel pressurized into accepting a compromise.

All I can say is persist. When you feel things are hopeless and people are refusing to listen, they may just have reached the point where a further push is all that's needed. In my case, the decision was overturned less than an hour before I had my treatment.

There are other channels of complaint, such as PALS, which I've mentioned before. If you are really making no headway, you could even seek legal advice, but I hope things are resolved before you need to do that.

My Story

The boost was completely different from the other radiotherapy treatments. For the main treatment, the radiotherapy machine would move in an arc around my body, so that my breast was being treated from many different angles. The boost used a different sort of radiation—electrons—and the machine stayed still above my breast, directing the radiation onto a specific area only. An electron beam is less penetrating than X-rays, so it's less likely to damage areas further in, such as my lungs.

The radiographer lined up the electron beam to the new felt-tip circle on my breast and disappeared behind a screen to give me the first dose.

Only four more treatments left, thank God.

The next day I was due to see Bronwen. On a whim I bought her a box of chocolates. She'd been such an angel, quietly watching over the radiation effects on my right breast, gently warning me of what would happen next and how to deal with it as well as helping my left breast wound to heal.

'Hello Kathleen, how're you doing? How's the radiotherapy going?' She greeted me with her usual smile.

'OK. My breast is a bit red and sore, and under my arm too, but otherwise it's fine. Dr. Ernest moved the boost area and I feel a lot happier now.'

'Oh, I'm so pleased.' She smiled. 'Right, the wound is healing steadily, but it'll take a few more weeks. Remember, don't force the dressing in. Just pack it lightly and let it close up. It's your last week of radiotherapy so just continue dressing it at home, but do call me or come in if you need to.'

What? Her words were like a mini-explosion in my head. She didn't want to see me anymore?

I recovered myself. The wound wasn't infected and was healing, so of course there was no need for her to check it. But I felt as if someone had sneaked off with my safety net. I'd got quite used to coming to the hospital every day. I'd been doing it for the last four weeks, and before that I was there most weeks too. I had my own little system. A walk through the park, take-away lunch from the Japanese shop, coffee at the hospital WRVS, maybe a piece of their home-made cake if it'd been a stressful day. In some way all my responsibilities were on hold—work, everything—I had a sick note from God.

Now suddenly she was talking about stopping. No more visits—what was I going to do? I'd have to become accountable for my life again, was I ready for that? Crikey, I thought, I'm getting institutionalized.

'Oh yes, of course Bronwen, I'll call you if I have a problem. Thanks so much for all you've done. You've been a tower of strength. Here, I bought you some chocolates.' (Thank Goodness I'd bought these today. I hadn't realised it would be

185

my last visit).

'Oh, they're lovely! You didn't need to do that Kathleen. It's been a pleasure.'

I left in a bit of a daze and headed down the stairs for day two of my 'Boost'.

I didn't go straight home after my treatment. I was meeting my daughter for dinner after work.

'Hi Mickie, how's Ed?'

'He's fine. He's sent you that information on your i-phone that you wanted. There you go.' she handed me a couple of sheets of printed notes, 'So how's things going with you?'

I filled her in on the latest developments of the 'Boost saga' and she told me about her holiday plans. It was great just to chat and eat and laugh about silly things, instead of focusing on my treatment.

I got home late and went straight to bed.

Then, out of the blue it seemed, it was Friday, the last day of my radiotherapy. Those unbearable four weeks which had seemed to stretch forever had finally come to an end. How had that happened?

I brought in boxes of chocolates for the staff. Most of them had been amazing— warm, kind, welcoming. I told the smiley Receptionist to make sure he had some. I would miss his cheery welcome.

As I dashed round the corner towards my radiotherapy machine I crashed straight into Dr Peters.

'Oops, sorry Dr Peters. It's my last treatment today and I wasn't concentrating.'

He smiled, 'Yes, I know. I came down to look for you actually. How are you?'

'I'm OK. Getting there.' I was surprised by his comment, and couldn't think of anything particularly intelligent to say.

'I just wanted to check you were all right.' He paused, 'I'm really sorry I was away when you sent that email. I was literally at the top of a mountain and couldn't do much. Poor internet connection, but I think Dr Ernest sorted things out for you? I was genuinely concerned that you were so upset.'

'Yes he did, thank you. He'd clearly spent a lot of time looking into my case and discussing things with the radiologists, and he went through all the latest research with me. I appreciated that.'

Dr Peters looked relieved. He hesitated again, 'I know what you're going through. It's not easy.'

I smiled, 'Well, I better take these chocs to the guys and have my last treatment.'

'You'll make them fat,' he returned my smile.

I walked through to the waiting area, 'Hello Cathy, how are you? Here are some chocolates for you all.' I knew most of the radiographers by name now.

I walked through with her, stripped off, put on my last blue gown, lay down under the machine, undid the gown and let them position me. Then it was all over. I got dressed, dropped the gown into the large bin, and left.

My son phoned me on his way home from work, 'How're you feeling Mum? Any news?'

'I'm fine Joe. Just had my last radiotherapy. It'll feel a bit strange actually, not going into the hospital every day.'

'Nice though, Mum. When do you have to go back?'

'I've a final appointment with Dr Peters in about three weeks, then one with Mrs Grant about seven weeks after that, then that's it. Just yearly mammograms for the next five years.'

'That's great Mum. We should celebrate. Do you want to have lunch tomorrow? Charlotte said she wants to cook for you.'

'Great Joe. Charlotte's cooking is always a treat, thank you.'

When I got home, I unlocked my front door wearily. I took off my coat and walked up the stairs to the bathroom. I ripped off my jumper and bra in front of the mirror and looked at the burned skin over my right chest. The blue–black tattoos glared at me, ugly and defiant.

The skin was damaged and sore—small scrolls of dead skin delicately peeling from the thinned, reddened skin beneath.

I had a plan. I took a flannel and started rubbing at the two tattoos, harder and faster, more and more desperately. If I could rub away that delicate skin, maybe the tattoos would rub away with it.

After a while, I stopped and looked in the mirror. All I'd done was create two deep, red, sore craters, but the tattoos were as big and black as before.

'You'll never get rid of us. You're stuck with us forever,' they mocked me.

The tears came, slowly at first, then unstoppable. I stared in the mirror and howled. Not just for the tattoos, but for everything.

187

Summary:

The boost is a different sort of radiation, using an electron beam, given directly to where the tumour had been

It is best to maintain a collaborative relationship with the medical staff but sometimes it goes wrong

If you are not listened to, first escalate to the consultant; if you still don't receive satisfaction, contact the hospital CEO and/or put your concern in writing

You could also ask your GP for a referral to a new consultant

Most importantly - persist

It is important to be knowledgeable about your condition, ask for and keep copies of hospital letters

It can be a shock when your treatment suddenly ends, after months of intensive hospital visits

Further Information:

Breast Cancer Care	http://goo.gl/jg5ieB
NHS Choices	http://bit.ly/1K38ryJ
NHS Complaints Guide	http://bit.ly/1PS6qh8

Chapter 23

After the treatment is finished

My Story

Over the next few weeks, I gradually 'resumed normal service'. I was still tired after my radiotherapy, and the skin and muscle soreness and stiffness took a while to settle. I used lots of moisturizer, aloe vera and bio-oil, which my friend's daughter Sonia had bought me. Friends kept in contact and checked on me. My son phoned most days and my daughter kept in touch by msn. I met up with them and their other halves when I could. Phil was now settled in his new home and we spoke by telephone occasionally.

I restarted some of my hobbies—ballroom dancing and walking, and I was touched that people seemed genuinely pleased to see me back.

Gradually I started to get emails enquiring whether I could take on any work. I resisted for a while, I just couldn't deal with it, but gradually I took on small bits, which grew into bigger bits, and it was fine.

I had my post-radiotherapy check with Dr Peters and saw Bronwen on the same day. My wound had still not completely closed, but it was getting there and I only needed to cover it with a small piece of gauze now.

After seeing Bronwen, I went back to the bra shop. I'd been wearing sports bras since my operation, to provide support to my healing breasts. They had served me well, but as the wound on the left breast was healing and the radiotherapy burns and swelling on the right were settling I was ready to take another step towards normality.

'What are you looking for today?' the young red-haired girl asked, as she led me into the tiny cubicle and pulled the dark, patterned curtain across.

189

'Well, I've just been treated for breast cancer so my bra-size has changed and I need a bra-fitting. I better warn you, I've had surgery, and there's still a small wound on one side.' *I didn't want her fainting at the unexpected sight of my war-torn chest. As per my recent habit, I stripped to the waist in front of her.*

She stared at my scarred breasts, her face impassive and professional as she assessed what size I needed, 'OK, let me bring a few bras.'

She reappeared a few minutes later with a selection of rather sensible-looking beige and white bras. I tried them on. 'Yes this one fits well, and it's comfortable, but it isn't very ... pretty.'

The girl laughed, 'Oh, you want pretty, do you?'

'Yes. I want to look like a princess.' I laughed back.

'Let's see what we have in the princess department then.' she pulled the cubicle curtain aside and disappeared.

A bundle of different coloured bras appeared in the gap in the curtain, followed by the girl. 'Here we are, bras fit for a princess.'

And they were—pretty turquoise, pink, green, feminine and dainty. Yes, I wanted to feel like a woman again. I bought two.

A couple of months after finishing the radiotherapy I had a final sign-off appointment with Mrs Grant. She checked me herself. She seemed to have a good system for seeing new patients personally, seeing them again after their operation and then at the final visit, delegating to her team at other times. It was nice to see the boss, and she always seemed to be available if needed. After declaring all was well, she sent me to Monica, the Breast Care Nurse.

Monica explained the Open Access system to me. If I had any worries about my breast, my GP didn't need to write to Mrs Grant for an appointment, with all the associated delays. I simply telephoned Monica to discuss my concerns, and if appropriate, she would arrange an appointment directly for me.

'Now, you're already on tamoxifen aren't you Kathleen?'

'Yes. Miss Gomez actually started me on it when my operation was delayed, so I've been on it for about seven months.'

'OK, well keep on it. The oncologists will review your treatment next year. They may change you then to letrozole or one of the other aromatase inhibitors, depending on your menopausal situation.'

'OK, thanks Monica.'

'You're welcome. Well that's it. You'll need a mammogram here every year

for five years, then you need to slot back into the normal national screening programme. Here's your appointment for the first mammogram next year. Don't forget, if you're worried in the meantime, or feel any new lumps or anything else, just give me a call. You've got my number there, haven't you?'

'Yes, it's here.'

'Right, well hopefully we won't need to see you until next year's mammogram.'

I left, clutching the small bundle of papers she'd given me: advisory booklets, contact numbers, mammogram appointment card and so on.

So then I was on my own. I'd had intensive medical interactions for around nine months, but now I had nothing planned for a year, other than daily tamoxifen.

Tamoxifen would block my natural oestrogen. As my cancer had oestrogen receptors, tamoxifen would lower the chance of my cancer returning.

I was given it because I hadn't completed the menopause. After the menopause, oestrogen is produced in the fat tissue, not the ovaries, and a group of drugs called Aromatase Inhibitors (AIs) (anastrozole, letrozole or exemestane) are more effective. Recent studies (including a study called BIG 1-98, in around eight thousand post-menopausal women) have shown that AIs seem to be more effective than tamoxifen once women have completed their menopause.

It used to be recommended to take tamoxifen or an AI for two years after finishing treatment, but now studies have shown that five years is better. As more information becomes available, this period may increase.

The drugs do have side-effects, including menopausal symptoms, such as hot flushes. Tamoxifen also increases your chances of getting cancer of the uterus, and AIs can cause bone pain, osteoporosis and heart disease. In pre-menopausal women tamoxifen affects fertility, so if you are considering starting a family you need to talk to your doctor.

Although the overall benefit of these drugs is quite clear from the statistics, you need to know what the actual benefit is going to be in your individual case. If your risk of recurrence is low anyway, you may be talking about just a few percent actual improvement, in which case you need to decide whether you want to take a drug and suffer possible side-effects for five years. It may be worth it to you, but you need the facts in order to decide.

Obviously not everyone is as lucky as I was—some are not given a clean bill of health and sent on their way. If your cancer wasn't successfully removed, or has spread to other parts of the body, then you will need further follow-ups and probably further treatment.

Alternatively, some people will have had successful surgery, but because of the features of their particular cancer, the chance of it returning may be much higher. If any of this applies to you, your story will be quite different, although some of the further information at the end of this chapter may be helpful.

However, even if you have been told your outlook is excellent, you may still not feel the elation you should. Your life has been on hold since the day you found yourself in Cancer World. People may expect you to put all these issues behind you and pick up the pieces where you left off. The trouble is, you're not the same person that you were. You carry scars, and not just on your chest. You'll never be quite the same again, for good or bad.

Importantly, you may experience a sense of anticlimax and bewilderment when your treatment ends, coupled with a secret guilt that you're not feeling happy and grateful for its success. This is quite normal, and you may need help to get through it, regardless of whether other people in your life understand.

Some people will have a very supportive family and/or friends, but even then their network may expect that now everything is back to normal they will be too. This isn't an unreasonable assumption, but it isn't correct or realistic either.

On the other hand you may feel absolutely fine and wonder what I'm wittering on about, but the shock of the whole thing can creep up on you when you least expect it, maybe even months or years later. I don't mean to be a harbinger of doom. I'm just warning you in case it happens, and I'd like to assure you that it doesn't mean you are crazy, flaky, inadequate or anything else other than normal.

But in any case your cancer story may not be over either...

My Story

So I was pootling along, gradually getting my life back together and adjusting to being not quite so special (although a mention that I'd recently had cancer still provoked a pleasing degree of reverence and shock in most people). I'd been told to check my breasts regularly, but I have to be honest, I was far too busy living life to remember to do this systematically (I know, you'd think, after all I'd been through, and me being a doctor and all. Well it turns out I was more human than doctor, and a bit lackadaisical at that).

Then, around six months after my treatment had finished, despite my lack of vigilance, I noticed that my breast was a bit firmer and more nobbly than usual where the cancer had been.

Just a bit of post-radiation fibrosis maybe? But I knew not to ignore it, and after a few days of anxious checking, I started to feel two distinct lumps. I had to get it checked.

I phoned Monica, the Breast Care Nurse. She gave me an appointment for the following week.

I was scared. I'd truly believed I was cured—the monster had left the building. If it had come back, where would it all end? Where was my safety net?

Finally the appointment day came. I walked through the familiar doors into out-patients. The heat hit me after the cold outside. The first person I saw was the Smiley Receptionist from radiotherapy.

I walked up to the desk, 'Hello. Have you switched departments?' I greeted him.

For less than a second, confusion clouded his face, then the sunny smile broke through, and I felt the warmth, 'Oh I remember you—nice to see you again.'

'You too. I've an appointment at 2.30pm.'

'Ah yes, take a seat—you know where to go.' His smile was irrepressible and contagious, and I sat in the waiting room, grinning like I'd won a ticket to the theatre, rather than an appointment with my favourite cancer specialist.

Then Bronwen walked by. In my excitement I stood up and called out, 'Hello Bronwen.' As I shouted, it occurred to me that she'd had literally hundreds of people through her care since I was last here, many more memorable than me. Why should she remember me?

I needn't have worried. She started, turned, then smiled, 'Kathleen, how nice to see you. How are things? Well, I say nice, but obviously I'd rather not see you back here. Is everything OK?'

'I've found another lump Bronwyn, but hopefully nothing to worry about.'

'Oh dear, well, fingers crossed. It's Dr. Middle in the clinic today. She's lovely. Not long to wait.'

I sat down, and after a few minutes a nurse called me into the consulting room.

193

A new face greeted me, 'Hello, I'm Dr. Middle. I gather you've found a lump?'

'Yes, it's hard to say how long it's actually been there, because my breast was a bit hard and lumpy anyway after the radiotherapy, but I do think there's a couple of definite lumps.'

'OK, well best if I take a look.'

I stripped to the waist and lay on the small couch. I'd rather got out of the habit, but the thin paper against my skin soon felt familiar again.

Dr. Middle started feeling my breast. Her relaxed demeanour calmed me. I imagined her thinking, oh yes, another routine lumpy breast. Examine and reassure. Too soon after her op to be anything worrisome.

But then I sensed a change in her. Her hand slowed as it moved over the lumps, and she seemed pensive. After what seemed a long time, she walked away from the couch and invited me to dress and sit down.

'Yes, there are definitely two lumps there. I'd like you to have an ultrasound scan. Take this form and pop along to the X-ray department. Come back here when you're finished. Just let the nurse know you're back.'

I walked down to the radiology department. I felt partly relieved that she'd found the lumps (I didn't want to look like a paranoid idiot), and partly terrified. I'd a heavy feeling in my stomach—not panic, but prepared for bad news.

When I got to X-ray, I handed in the form and sat and waited. I felt calm but edgy. I started to imagine what would happen if my cancer had come back. I still hadn't sorted out my finances, so back to square one on the inheritance tax front. I'd have to tell my kids the bad news, just as they'd started to relax about the whole thing. All the things I'd started doing—my dancing, walking—all of that would be put back on hold again. And, I didn't want to think about it, but my outlook was likely to be worse than the first time around if I did have a recurrence.

'Kathleen Thompson?' The radiographer's call broke into my thoughts.

I followed her into the waiting area with the inevitable pile of blue gowns and small cubicles. As instructed, I got changed and walked into the ultrasound room, where the radiologist was waiting, and lay down.

The radiologist was a middle-aged man. He reminded me of the doctor who'd done my first ultrasound and taken the first biopsy—almost exactly a year ago.

'Hello, well you know what's going to happen, I'm sure.' His smile was gentle. 'I just need to examine these lumps with the ultrasound, and then we'll go from there. So first can you point them out to me?'

I obliged and, using the ultrasound probe and the usual blob of gel, he found them on his small monitor.

He stared for a few minutes then spoke quietly to the radiographer, 'I'll need to try to aspirate these.' I could tell he wasn't happy.

Turning to me he spoke in a more normal voice, 'I think the best thing is to stick a needle into these two lumps and see what comes out. If there's fluid, we'll send it off to the lab. If there isn't, I may need to go in and take a biopsy.' He looked into my eyes as he spoke.

Like the first radiologist, he seemed to be sending me courage. He didn't need to. I'd picked up that there was a concern, but I was ready for it this time. Like a soldier preparing for battle, I knew the score. It wasn't great, but I could deal with it all again if I had to do.

He numbed my skin, but this time instead of a biopsy needle, he pushed an ordinary needle attached to a syringe into my breast, all the while looking at his monitor to guide the needle into the lump.

He started to pull back on the plunger. He glanced at the fluid in the syringe then let his breath out loudly and beamed at me, indicting the syringe with his eyes for me to see. I looked—the syringe was filling with very dark blood.

'Old blood—it must have been a haematoma left from your operation. I don't even have to send that to the lab.' he pulled out the syringe and needle from my breast and practically flung them into the metal kidney dish on the trolley.

I was thrilled, relieved and actually quite touched by his reaction. He didn't know me, and yet he couldn't have seemed happier if I'd had been his mother (not that I was old enough, I should point out).

'OK, let's aspirate the other one now. I'm less worried about that one. I suspect it's just a bit of fat necrosis.'

As he pulled on the second syringe, it filled with a milky liquid, 'Yep, fat necrosis. Just dead fat. Hopefully now I've emptied them, the lumps will disappear. They may fill up again, but it's nothing to worry about.'

He seemed so happy I half-expected him to reach into the instrument trolley and bring out a half bottle of Bolly and three glasses (sadly he didn't).

My head was swimming. My eyes were a little damp—but for such different reasons from last time.

I went back to the outpatients and announced the good news to Dr Middle. She looked genuinely delighted too. My lumps had clearly resembled cancer from their reactions. I couldn't believe I'd been spared.

I left the hospital and phoned my son. He'd left work and was due at the station at about the same time as I would get there. I arranged to meet him. As I walked there I phoned my daughter and told her the good news. 'That's brilliant Mum, thanks for letting me know. Are you going to celebrate?'

When I got to the station I asked my son if we could go for a drink.

'Sure Mum, my treat, what would you like?'

'Actually I'd like a glass of prosecco please, Joe.'

'Of course, Mum.'

It tasted so good.

A month later I had a telephone conversation with the Department of Genetics. Earlier I'd asked about my daughter's risk of breast cancer, as several members of my family had also had the disease. I'd been told that it was unlikely, as my relatives were all relatively old when they'd developed the cancer. However, my blood had been tested for BRCA 1 and BRCA 2 genes, genes known to be associated with a high risk of breast cancer. The phone call was to let me know that I didn't possess these genes. This was more good news.

BRCA 1 and BRCA 2 genes are associated with a very high risk of breast and ovarian cancer in women, and prostate cancer and breast cancer in men, as well as an increased risk of pancreatic cancer in both sexes. If you are tested and found to have these genes, you and your family will be advised on your individual risks. Women found to have these genes have been known to have mastectomies before they develop cancer, as Angelina Jolie did. This is of course a personal decision.

My story

A few months later I had my first annual mammogram, which confirmed that the lumps I had found were not cancer.

Six months later I developed another new lump, which was also found to be fat necrosis. Much of the breast is composed of fat, and after radiotherapy small areas of this fatty tissue can die. This can feel like a lump. I remembered Miss Gomez's original warning about needing repeated checks and biopsies as lumps like this could appear. Although I was becoming more relaxed about them, they always had to be checked out—just in case.

I had one further scare, around two years after my treatment ended—another lump, but this time I also had severe pain in my lumbar spine, which lasted for several months. Dr Middle was confident that the pain was a red herring, but she knew I was worrying in case the cancer had come back and had gone to my bones, so she arranged a bone scan.

I could tell something was wrong when I had the scan. The radiographer, who had seemed very bored when she'd started the scan, suddenly became extremely interested in whether I'd had any problems with my lumbar spine. She obviously hadn't noticed that back pain was the reason for my referral.

I interpreted (correctly as it turned out) that her sudden interest related to what she'd seen on my bone scan. My worst fears seemed to be coming true. If the cancer had spread to my bones, it was very serious.

I then had my spine X-rayed to see whether the abnormality on the bone scan was due to cancer or just arthritis. Let's just say I have never been so pleased to learn that I had some osteoarthritis in my spine.

Since then—so far so good. But my case is not unusual. Various things can appear after cancer, all of which need checking. You shouldn't ignore them, and frankly most people are inclined to assume the worst whenever they find a new breast lump or have an odd pain somewhere. It's hardly surprising. As such, the Open Access system is extremely practical and helpful.

Summary:

An Open Access Policy allows patients to contact their hospital directly for anything relating to their cancer treatment for a period of time after their treatment finishes

If the cancer has oestrogen receptors, treatment to block these will probably be prescribed for 5 years or longer—usually either tamoxifen or an aromatase inhibitor

New lumps may appear in your breasts. They should always be taken seriously, but may be fat necrosis due to the radiotherapy, and can appear long after the treatment is finished.

It may take you a long time to recover psychologically from cancer, and the reaction may hit you much later.

Some people have a genetic susceptibility to breast cancer and other cancers, particularly if they have a BRCA 1 or BRCA 2 gene, in which case genetic counselling for the family is important

Further Information:

BreastCancer.org   http://goo.gl/IIguCN

Dr Susan Love's Breast Book: S M Love with K Lindsey – Da Capo

BreastCancer.org	http://goo.gl/ZQcdFO
Macmillan Cancer Support	http://goo.gl/rlqtUZ
Cancer Research UK	http://goo.gl/bJhX6Y
Breast Cancer Care	http://goo.gl/HHxgH6
National Cancer Institute	http://goo.gl/IJclBi
NICE	http://goo.gl/rQOT7B

Book: The Breast Cancer Book by V. Sampson and D Fenlon published Vermilion 2000

Chapter 24

What if the cancer comes back?

Breast cancer goes away for good in many people, but not everyone. If it's going to return it's usually within two years. However a few people suffer a recurrence many years later.

The cancer can reappear in different ways. Sometimes it can be found in the skin near the site of the original tumour—called a local recurrence, usually treatable by surgery or radiotherapy. Alternatively it may appear in the lymph nodes near the tumour site; this is called a regional recurrence.

If it appears in another part of the body, such as your bones, lung, liver or even brain it is called secondary cancer, and is more serious. However, there are still many treatment options even with secondary breast cancer, and some people can live for many years with it. The difference is that you will be *living with* cancer, as, usually, secondary breast cancer cannot be eradicated completely, at least at the time of writing.

Treatment may be chemotherapy or radiotherapy or hormonal therapy, such as tamoxifen. There are various new drugs which specifically target tumour cells wherever they are, and sometimes some of the cancer can be removed surgically. In this way your cancer can be controlled for a long time.

New drugs—and new ways of using old drugs—are constantly being studied, and you may be asked if you want to take part in a clinical trial. Consider this possibility carefully. It may or may not be right for you, but sometimes you can gain a lot from the opportunity.

It would be wrong to ignore the fact that for some people, the cancer recurrence is very serious, and they will not be expected to live for long. This brings a whole series of issues, both emotional and practical—telling your

199

family and friends, your children, making arrangements for their continuing care, financial security, accepting your impending death, the list goes on.

There are many fears associated with knowing that your cancer is unlikely to go away. Fear of death itself; fear of pain; fear of being a burden; fear of isolation (no one can really understand); fear of leaving your partner/children/friends forever; fear of what happens when you die; fear of not finishing important things in your life.

You may not believe it, but many of these fears can be addressed, and may even go away completely with the right help and knowledge. Counselling can help, as can discussing your future care with your doctor; there are usually ways to deal with pain, and if you understand what can be done, this may help you deal with your fear. Many people with terminal illness do learn to accept death, and it becomes less frightening.

Leaving children behind is always associated with anguish. There are some positive things you can do in regard to this—letters from you for them to open at certain ages, memory boxes, and so on.

If you want to look into the spiritual side of death more, depending on your core beliefs, you may find The Tibetan Book of Living and Dying helpful.

Most people will need professional support both for themselves and their loved ones during this time, and various organisations, including the cancer charities can be helpful. I would recommend Val Sampson and Debbie Fenlon's book as well worth reading should you be touched by this situation.

Besides experimental drugs, you may be tempted by various alternative therapies at this point, including special diets. I make no recommendations for or against these. In most cases there have been no large-scale clinical trials, but that doesn't necessarily mean they won't work. You need to assess alternative treatments carefully though, as there are some cancer 'cures' which may have no benefit and may be harmful. I provide guidance on how to approach alternative therapies in a subsequent chapter.

Summary:

If breast cancer recurs it usually does so within 2 years, but it can recur after many years too.
It is most serious if it appears somewhere in the body away from the original tumour, such as the lungs or bones—this is secondary cancer. In this case you will probably need to live with the cancer rather than hoping for cure
Treatment can still help you
Experimental new therapies may be an option
You may consider various alternative therapies. That is a personal decision

Further Information:

Macmillan Cancer Support   http://goo.gl/1uBQkI
Breast Cancer Care   http://goo.gl/a82Jk9
Cancer Research UK   http://goo.gl/UM1VgL

Book: The Breast Cancer Book by V. Sampson and D Fenlon published Vermilion 2000

The Tibetan Book of Living and Dying by Sogyal Rinpoche

Chapter 25

Breast cancer in men

Men do get breast cancer, but much less frequently than women, probably because they only have a small amount of breast tissue. They also have less natural oestrogen than women, and more testosterone, which counteracts the oestrogen.

A man may be more likely to get breast cancer if his natural oestrogens are raised, if he is overweight or has liver disease.

Some genetic conditions predispose men to breast cancer, such as possessing the BRCA 2 gene (see earlier chapter), or Klinefelter's syndrome (having an extra X chromosome). Radiation exposure may sometimes be a cause too.

If a man feels any lumps under or around his nipple, anywhere in or near the chest or under his arm, he should have them checked. Likewise any nipple changes such as a discharge, or changes in shape, or hardness or soreness, should be discussed with a doctor. This is important, because men with breast cancer usually don't seek medical help until very late on, and by then their outlook is less favourable.

Usually breast cancer in men occurs in the over-sixties, but not exclusively, so never dismiss any signs.

It's no fun having breast cancer, for anyone—but I suspect it's harder for a man. Besides the embarrassment of having what is considered a women's illness, it must be difficult to attend patient support groups when you're the only man and everyone assumes you've got lost looking for the car maintenance class.

Currently there are only around 350 men diagnosed per year in the UK, and even some breast cancer centres have relatively little experience with male breast cancer, so it is probably best to go to a large specialist unit.

Although the treatment is very similar to the treatment for women, Breast Cancer Care have produced a series of booklets specifically for men which can be downloaded for free from their website.

Summary:

350 men per year in UK are diagnosed with breast cancer
Predisposing factors include raised oestrogen levels, genetic conditions and
radiation exposure
Check out any lumps in the vicinity of your breast or under the arm, or any
changes to, or discharges from, your nipple

Further Information:

Cancer Research UK	http://goo.gl/jTSNjj
NHS Choices	http://bit.ly/1MJlgjw
Breast Cancer Care	http://goo.gl/2NpDnm

Chapter 26

Complimentary medicine

I use the word 'complimentary' rather than 'alternative'. Many healing systems have been developed around the world since ancient times, and it would seem foolish to ignore all the wisdom and knowledge they contain. Equally, why deny yourself conventional medicine? Why choose? Take the best of everything — because, as a well-known shampoo company keeps reminding everyone, you're worth it.

Conventional medicine has made great inroads into the treatment of many cancers. The Cancer UK website tells us that cancer survival in the UK has doubled over the last forty years. This isn't all due to new therapies, but some of it is.

However, there are many established complimentary medicines which are definitely worth exploring to use alongside conventional medicine. I can't possibly name all of them but I have personally used Ayurveda, acupuncture, spiritual/Reiki healing, reflexology and meditation and I have found benefit in all of these.

My understanding of Eastern health systems such as Chinese medicine and Indian Ayurvedic medicine is that they work on the premise that illness results when the body, spirit and mind are out of balance. They focus on the person as a whole and ask why we got cancer in the first place? Addressing the cause could affect our current cancer and reduce our risk of further cancers.

Ayurveda practitioners use herbal medicines, but they also prescribe diet and exercise. Some traditional ayurvedic medicines are being tested in clinical trials, such as at the Dhanwanthari Centre in Kerala, India. This is exciting, as there are copious herbal remedies used by the tribal people in the rainforests of Kerala. Local Indians often consult tribal experts in addition to doctors practicing conventional western medicine. Many modern medicines originated from plants in the first place, and if rainforest plants were studied in clinical trials, a huge number of potentially effective medicines could become available.

A word of caution; herbal treatments can contain powerful active ingredients, which may interact with conventional medicines. If you do try herbal medicines, you must let your doctor know and make sure it's safe to combine it with your other medicines.

Penny Brohn Cancer Care, also known as the Bristol Approach, is based in Bristol but offers courses locally too. The centre was started by Penny, who had breast cancer, and her friend, Pat. They recognised that people with cancer needed more than just medical treatment. The centre offers advice and courses on nutrition, lifestyle and more. They have a useful website, and you may consider attending one of their courses.

You may want to try spiritual healing or Reiki healing. The Harry Edwards Healing Sanctuary near Guildford is a beautiful, peaceful place. You can wander around the lovely grounds and receive spiritual healing if you wish. You can also find Spiritual or Reiki healers locally and through Spiritualist churches. I found it very helpful.

There are many other complimentary therapies such as homeopathy, hypnotherapy and massage. Different therapies help different people. These treatment systems are generally compatible with conventional medicine, but I would strongly caution against using them *instead* of conventional medicine. Conventional medicine may not be perfect, but it has been well-tested and has proven efficacy and any safety issues are well-understood. This is often not the case for alternative treatments.

There are numerous 'anti-cancer' dietary treatments promoted on the internet. Some appear to have little or no scientific verification (see next chapter), and some are difficult to follow and/or preclude many foodstuffs which are generally considered healthy. They are of particular concern when their proponents discourage people from using conventional cancer therapy.

One dietary therapy which deserves mention is the Gerson Therapy, developed by Dr Max Gerson. The regime involves frequent juicing of organic vegetables and fruit, low protein, low sodium and mainly plant-based raw foods, coffee enemas, and various supplements such as iodine, pancreatic enzymes, thyroxine and liver extracts, amongst other things. It is claimed that it 'allows the body to heal itself'.

My personal view is that some aspects of Gerson therapy do have merits. Providing a constant supply of micronutrients and antioxidants through high intake of organic fresh fruit and vegetables, and avoiding foodstuffs which are harmful, such as processed food, sugar, sweets, cakes, and soft drinks, is consistent with current recommendations on a healthy diet. However many other healthy foods are excluded, including avocados, berries, nuts, green tea.

I cannot endorse or censure Gerson Therapy. I simply don't have enough information to do either. There are very few published studies, and most are in small numbers of patients, or case reports, which do not provide the statistical data necessary to reach an objective conclusion.

The Gerson Institute did conduct a study in 153 patients with melanoma in 1995. This was a retrospective study, and relied on comparisons with data from other studies. Results from these types of study designs are generally less reliable than those from studies designed in accordance with the requirements for regulatory drug approval (see next chapter). In addition, 96 of the original 249 patients were excluded from the analysis, 53 because they were lost to follow-up. Such a high percentage of exclusions is a concern with regard to the reliability of the study results.

Nevertheless, the data are interesting, and further, controlled, prospective studies of this therapy are essential if it is to be adequately assessed for benefit in people with cancer.

There are numerous other alternative treatments available on the internet. Many don't have a rational scientific basis, and while I can't tell you categorically that they don't work, I would advise you to be open-minded but discerning—and remember, *caveat emptor*; buyer beware.

Summary:

Complimentary treatments can be helpful
Consider using them with conventional medicine, not instead of— although it is your choice
Their effectiveness usually hasn't been tested in rigorous scientific studies, as happens with conventional drugs, but this doesn't necessarily mean they don't work. All it means is that there is less evidence
Some treatments promoted on the internet may be untested, unscientific and even dangerous. Other treatments may be genuine. 'Pseudo-science' can be convincing. There are some clues, but unless you have scientific training it can be difficult to be sure. Be wary and seek expert opinions to assess authenticity and reliability of scientific claims

Further Information:

What is Ayurveda?	http://goo.gl/9nCVbR
Dhanwanthari Vaidyasala	http://goo.gl/9Bp7oM
Penny Brohn Cancer Care	http://goo.gl/yJQOkI
Breast Cancer Care	http://goo.gl/gfO1qr
Cancer Research UK	http://goo.gl/wkD43o
NCBI	http://goo.gl/NOizSk

Chapter 27

How to do your own research

When I was a young doctor, I would read the latest research in journals in my medical library. The papers had been written many months prior to publication, and the actual study would have finished maybe a year earlier. Without access to a specialist library, it was even harder to access such information.

Now, with a little help from Mr Google, anyone can obtain up-to-date information on pretty much anything within seconds. Particularly useful sources include Medline, scientific library websites and individual journal websites.

But how do we know whether the information is genuine, rational, unbiased or reliable? The problem is that anyone can post anything on the internet—there's no truth or accuracy filter. Consequently there are many unsubstantiated claims, uninformed opinions and just plain lies or misconceptions.

So how do we sift out the genuine grains of knowledge from the unreliable chaff?

If you have cancer, particularly if your cancer has a poor outlook, it's very tempting to grab any lifeboat-shaped straw, no matter how tenuous. It has to be your decision what you choose to believe, but in this chapter I will provide some tools to help you assess what you read.

First I will talk about the types of information you will find on the internet. Then I will explain the main types of studies you are likely to read about, and their strengths and pitfalls. I will explain how studies on patients (clinical trials) should be conducted. It is important to understand the principles of a well-conducted study in order to recognize a poor one in which the results may be less reliable. Finally I will offer an example of internet claims which I consider misleading—again to help you recognize similar cases. So, here goes.

You will be exposed to three main groups of information:

1. 'Conventional medical thinking'—in the form of charity booklets (such as those produced by Breast Cancer Care and Macmillan), textbooks, research publications and orthodox medical websites for example.

2. Established alternative therapies such as Ayurvedic medicine and Chinese medicine. It's unusual for these to have gone through a full programme of clinical trials, although some Ayurvedic treatments are currently being tested. This doesn't necessarily mean they don't work, and some have been developed over many hundreds or even thousands of years, so don't dismiss them out of hand.

3. Claims which are not based on established medical practice, western or otherwise. Some of these may be supported by reliable research, others may sound very convincing but are based on small, badly designed trials with unreliable data—or even no studies at all.

There are three main types of studies which you may encounter.

1. 'Laboratory studies'
Either animal or test-tube studies. These are required by regulatory authorities and are often done before a drug is tested in people. The ethics of animal experimentation are beyond the scope of this book.

The results *may* predict how a drug will perform. However, often very high doses are tested in animals, sometimes much higher than could safely be dosed to humans; humans and animals sometimes respond differently; test-tube studies are even further removed, and assume that humans will be exposed to all the drug, whereas often our body breaks it down into different chemicals, which may have different effects. Consequently, sometimes no benefit is seen when humans are subsequently studied after either test-tube or animal studies.

These studies can be useful screening processes for new drugs, helping to pick potentially useful drugs out of many hundreds of chemicals tested.

However, one shouldn't get too excited about a newspaper headline for a new cancer cure if it was based on one study in thirty mice. It makes good press, but is merely an indication that a substance may be worth testing further.

2. Epidemiological studies

These are 'hands-off' studies which just observe large groups of people. They're particularly useful for finding how life-style affects illness. For instance, smoking causes lung cancer. It may seem obvious now, but people only began to suspect this in the 1940s, and most doctors didn't believe it until epidemiological studies in the 1940s and 50s proved the link.

In these studies it is key to distinguish *association* from *causation*. As an example, Chinese people eat a lot of rice. They generally have black hair. Does this mean that eating rice causes black hair? No, it's just coincidence. Black hair and eating rice are both *associated* with being Chinese, but eating rice does not *cause* black hair.

Well-designed studies use complex statistical techniques to avoid making incorrect assumptions about causation, while poorly-designed studies often don't. This can result in serious misinterpretations.

Epidemiology can be used to study the influence of diet on cancer. It's difficult to isolate one aspect of the diet; we can't just feed people one thing for, say two years, to see whether they get cancer or not. However, populations with very stable diets have been studied, for example in *The China Study* by T. Colin Campbell and colleagues—of which more later.

3. Clinical Trials

Clinical trials are carefully controlled studies in humans. A large number of these must be completed to demonstrate that a licensed medicine works and is safe, before it can to be sold.

There are different laws for herbal preparations. Some traditional herbal treatments carry a Traditional Herbal registration (THR) registration mark. This guarantees the product quality, but they haven't undergone all the clinical trials and other tests of a licensed medicine. They can only claim to work for minor conditions, not requiring medical supervision.

Some non-pharmaceutical 'cures' are sold as food-stuffs or dietary supplements for example, and are not approved medicines or herbal products. They may not have been tested for benefit at all.

I am going to talk about clinical trials in detail, as you will find the words 'evidence from studies' quoted on the internet time after time to support cancer cure claims. It is important to be able to recognize whether this 'evidence' is reliable.

A drug developed by a pharmaceutical company undergoes several years of laboratory testing before it is ever given to a human being. By then, much is known about its chemical make-up, how it works, how the body breaks it down and eliminates it, and likely beneficial effect and possible side-effects. Many thousands of potential drugs never even make it past this point.

When the testing eventually indicates that it is safe, the drug will go through a large programme of clinical trials. A small clinical trial is usually performed first, followed by larger studies in different types of patients, testing different doses or treatment durations—all building up comprehensive information about how it can help people.

Regulatory authorities and ethical committees for Europe, USA and elsewhere check the study design before a clinical trial can proceed. They make sure that patients are not put at risk, and that the study design is sensible and scientifically sound.

The design of the study will vary, but there are some important principles which should apply to all studies to ensure that the results are scientifically valid. These include the following:

1. Placebo comparison

People can influence trial results by their beliefs. Both doctor and patient may think a patient is improving if they believe the drug is effective. This is called the 'placebo effect'. Sometimes even patient's blood tests improve, which just shows how powerful the effect can be.

This is natural and normal, and doesn't imply that either the patient or the doctor is feeble-minded or unduly suggestible.

For this reason, most clinical trials will include an extra group of patients who are given a placebo (a dummy drug). A computer will decide who gets the real drug, and nobody directly involved in the trial knows who has received what. In this way no one can inadvertently bias the results.

Sometimes it isn't possible to have a placebo group, but if at all possible one is included. Sometimes the new drug is tested against an established drug, either in addition to, or in place of a placebo. If you find claims on the internet based on studies which didn't have a placebo group, without a good reason, you should be cautious.

2. A pre-specified primary endpoint

The investigators must decide in advance exactly how they are going to run the study. This will be written down in a study protocol. Importantly, they must state how they will decide whether the drug has worked; this is called the primary endpoint. For example, if they are studying the common cold, the primary endpoint could be improving runny noses. If runny noses didn't improve, the investigators can't change their minds when they get the results and say "well, it didn't work in runny noses but it had a good effect on sneezing." The drug would have failed in that study, because the primary endpoint was not met.

The reason for this is that if you trawl through all possible effects that have improved more in the treated group, you will eventually find one—which may well have occurred by chance—and if you pick this out and ignore all the other effects, you may wrongly assume that the drug has worked. This is something to watch out for in *non-regulated* studies, posted on the internet.

The researchers may decide to do another study with sneezing as the primary endpoint—that's fine, but then they *must* use sneezing as the measure of success, and can't switch back to runny noses if the results look better for this in the new study.

3. The study must have enough patients (powering)

As an extreme example, if a study only had two patients, and one received the drug and the other the placebo, and if the patient on the drug improved and the other didn't, you could say that 100% (all) of the patients who took the drug improved. Obviously, this could just have been chance, and results based on one patient are neither impressive nor convincing.

However if there were a hundred patients in each group, and eighty taking the real drug improved, compared to only ten taking the placebo, then the effect is more likely to be genuine.

For regulated studies, statisticians do complex calculations to ensure that studies are adequately powered—meaning that there are enough patients give a reliable result. Poorly designed studies may be based on too few patients to give meaningful results.

4. Control of the types of patients

The patients studied should be pre-defined to avoid confounding factors. In the common cold trial, if any patients happened to have hayfever then they may get a runny nose due to that, rather than their cold. This will mask any benefit of the drug on their cold. So allowing patients with hayfever to take part in this study would just confuse the findings. Some of these restrictions may be relaxed in later, larger studies.

It is also important that the characteristics of the patients to be studied are decided before any study results are available. In retrospective studies, where the data is already known, there is a potential risk of selecting the patient groups who gave the desired results, and disregarding other groups.

5. Accountability and audit

Study data should be carefully checked and audited to make sure that nobody has 'cheated' (inventing participants, falsifying data). Once such concerns have been addressed and satisfied, the results are written up as a report and submitted to a scientific journal for publication. Here the results will be reviewed by experts, and only accepted for publication if the study is considered scientifically valid.

Pharmaceutical drug studies have to follow all these procedures. If studies didn't include all these elements, companies could claim beneficial effects on the basis of results which were flawed or hadn't been adequately proven. The regulatory authorities would not approve the sale of such drugs.

The design and results of all clinical trials used to approve drugs are available on the European Medicines Agency (EMA) and FDA websites, so you can read for yourself what studies have been done and what results were obtained.

This gives you an idea of the scientific standards required to prove that a drug works and has acceptable levels of safety. Despite the rigour, these tests are still not 100% foolproof, and side-effects sometimes don't become apparent until after a drug has been approved and many thousands of patients have been treated with it. To address this, the regulatory authorities have systems to detect dangerous side-effects post-marketing, and if necessary, withdraw the drug from sale.

In contrast agents, which are not classed as drugs including some herbal and homeopathic preparations, are not required to undergo any such testing. This doesn't mean they won't work, and they may have been tested in other well-designed clinical trials. However, it's unlikely that they will have been tested on as many patients, or to such a high degree as for most approved drugs.

There are many books that claim to tell you how to beat cancer. If a book backs up its statements by referencing numerous publications from well-respected medical journals, it should give you more confidence.

However, even the devil can cite scripture, and sometimes small parts of a publication (maybe just one sentence) are taken out of context and then used to 'support' wild statements. How can you tell? Well it's difficult to be certain without going back to the original article, but you can get an idea by looking at the title of the reference and judging whether the quotation seems to reflect the actual publication. If not, it may well be a statement taken out of context. Equally, if the majority of the references are from little known or irrelevant journals, such as the Annals of Outer Mongolian Fishing Boats, you may start to suspect the quality of the quoted study.

Respected researchers would always aim to have their results published in the most prestigious medical journal possible. If you're not sure whether a journal is high quality, you can check its Impact Factor. It isn't foolproof, but a journal with a high impact factor is generally reputable.

Anyone can start a journal, and some bogus journals have misleading names implying that they are legitimate publications. You can always ask your GP or consultant's opinion if you are unsure.

One example of an alternative cancer treatment you may encounter is the alkaline diet. This is promoted on many internet websites. I would like to use this as an example of how scientifically incorrect statements may be misleading and harmful.

Rationales given by some websites for the alkaline diet appear to be based on the following assumptions:

1. Cancers tend to grow in an acid environment.
2. If foods are burned, some produce a residue which is acidic, and some an alkaline residue. These foods are referred to as 'acidic' and 'alkaline' foods respectively.

3. Eating 'alkaline' foods and avoiding 'acidic' foods raises the pH within the body. This creates an alkaline environment around cancer cells and they die.

In my opinion, this rationale is flawed for two major reasons. Firstly, the acidic or alkaline status of a food may change after burning. Lemons are classed as 'alkaline' based on their residue, and yet we all know that lemon juice is acidic.

Secondly, the healthy body regulates blood pH within a very narrow, slightly alkaline range of 7.35-7.45, using the lungs and kidneys. Breathing rate controls pH through removal of carbon dioxide, and the kidneys regulate how much acid or alkali is lost in the urine. If the pH does stray outside this tight range, the person will quickly become quite ill. So pH around a cancer cannot be significantly changed by diet, unless the lungs and/or kidneys are not working properly.

Much of the alkaline diet includes fresh fruit and vegetables and excludes processed foods and sugar-based products and any benefits probably relate to discouraging unhealthy foods. However, many versions of this diet also exclude important healthy foods, such as lentils, olives, squash, blueberries, barley, oats, quinoa, spelt, numerous beans, dairy products, some nuts, many meats and fish, and many oils including flax oil.

Further claims made by some advocates of this diet, such as, two foods which are alkaline when eaten separately may become acidic when eaten together doesn't make any scientific sense to me.

Some promoters of this diet recommend a regular intake of bicarbonate of soda as an anti-cancer therapy. As explained above, taking bicarbonate will not significantly affect the acidity around a tumour, except in the presence of kidney disease, when taking large doses of bicarbonate would be very dangerous. I cannot see any justification for this advice.

I use this as an example of how something can sound very scientific and convincing when in fact it is flawed. Be wary of internet-based information unless you fully understand the science behind it.

I would just like to add another cautionary word about another product that pervades the anti-cancer internet sites. It is known as Amygdalin, vitamin B17, or in its chemically modified version, Laetrile. Amygdalin is found in different fruit pits including apricot kernels, peach stones and bitter almonds, plus in certain plants, and many people strongly believe that it can be used to treat cancer. Laetrile may or may not work, but, to date, many clinical studies have shown no benefit and it has not gone through the rigorous testing required by regulatory authorities. The evidence is insufficient to confirm firstly whether it works at all and secondly what constitutes an effective or a safe dose. Laetrile contains cyanide, which can be released by gut enzymes and bacteria, leading to very variable, and sometimes dangerously high cyanide levels in the blood and there have been reports of cyanide poisoning, sometimes fatal, with its use. It is not available legally as a medicine in the UK for these reasons. Some people advocate obtaining amygdalin or laetrile from abroad, or even eating apricot kernels directly, or crushed. Using any of these unregulated preparations will give you no guarantee of dose or product quality, and as such is potentially very dangerous. The Sloan-Kettering Cancer Center in USA has given, in my opinion, a balanced summary on Laetrile (see Further Information below).

Having said all this, there is another side. The medical establishment tends to be conservative, for good reasons. It's important to test any potential new cancer treatment rigorously, before dosing people. However, the downside is that sometimes inspired babies do get thrown out with the research bath water too. Important new ideas have sometimes been resisted and even ridiculed by conventional medicine for many years.

For example, when I was a young doctor, we believed that peptic ulcers and gastritis were caused by too much stomach acid. So patients underwent major operations, cutting the vagus nerve and widening the stomach exit, in order to reduce stomach acid.

Then two scientists, Marshall and Warren, discovered that in fact the culprit was a bacterium called Helicobacter pylori—H. pylori to its friends. But nobody would believe them. Eventually Marshall, in desperation, had a stomach biopsy and then swallowed a large quantity of H. pylori to give himself acute gastritis. Only then did the medical world accept their findings. Nowadays, these conditions are treated by a simple course of antibiotics to kill the H. pylori.

So you can see that treatment is a tricky path to follow. Either you take the ultra-conservative route and risk missing some innovative cancer treatment, or you read everything on the internet, and risk being taken in by what may be well-meaning cranks. All you can do is assess the information and the source as well as you can and make your own decision. Consult the advice of experts, but keep an open mind too.

Summary:

There is no quality filter for the infinite information available on the internet
There are three main types of cancer studies you may encounter:
1. **Laboratory studies** (animal or 'test-tube') — don't necessarily predict human effect
2. **Epidemiological** (observational) studies — useful to assess lifestyle/diet on cancer
3. **Clinical trials** — must be well-designed to produce meaningful data.
Beware of 'journals' and websites with scientific-sounding names which make convincing-sounding claims — check they are legitimate
Remain open-minded to new ideas, but check them carefully

Further Information:

Breast Cancer UK	http://goo.gl/vuRDCN
Macmillan Cancer Support	http://goo.gl/kbWpcp
European Medicines Agency	http://goo.gl/5sbGoh
American Cancer Society	http://goo.gl/mFxJPo
CiteFactor	http://goo.gl/ijXvSz
National Cancer Institute	http://goo.gl/8Ooa4R

The China Study by T. Colin Campbell, BenBella Books Inc

PubMed (NCBI)	http://goo.gl/70Zw6r
Free Medical Journals	http://goo.gl/em4RM7
Cancer Research UK	http://goo.gl/BYdnjp
MSKCC	http://goo.gl/1dmEdh
PubMed Health (PDQ)	http://goo.gl/7CXd0o

Chapter 28

What can you do for yourself to combat cancer?

There's a lot more information on this topic than you may realise. There is mounting evidence that we can improve our chances against cancer and lead a generally healthy and more enjoyable life by making some simple life-style changes.

As I said before, cancer cells develop in all of our bodies on a very regular basis, just as we are regularly exposed to infections. But we don't all get cancer, just as we don't all succumb to pneumonia or meningitis. Most of the time our immune system deals with cancer cells and infections before we even know they're there, and it's only when this fails that we develop signs of disease.

So the answer is simple... isn't it? We need to increase the odds that our body will do its job and keep destroying the cancer cells before they take over. This means maintaining a strong immune system and reducing or at least weakening attacks on it—a basic principle of any conflict. We already follow these steps to protect ourselves from infection—things like washing our hands, keeping meat in the fridge, boosting our immunity with vaccinations and so on.

Another important and related anti-cancer strategy is to reduce inflammation in our bodies. Inflammation can be a good thing, it is the body's protective response to damage and to invasion by infections such as bacteria. It is how our immune system destroys and removes infective organisms and dead cells and promotes repair of damaged body tissues.

However, if cancer cells manage to avoid being discovered and dealt with by our immune system and are not destroyed, they can turn our inflammatory

220

response against us, helping them grow and spread. They do this in various ways, for example by using inflammatory activity to grow new blood vessels, which provide the tumour with a source of food and oxygen. This also means that our immune cells are occupied in maintaining this cancer-induced inflammation, and have less resources available to fight the cancer, or any infection that we may contract.

So, although short bursts of inflammation can be protective, long term inflammation is certainly not. In fact some chronic inflammatory illnesses are known to predispose us to cancer. Inflammatory bowel disease, for example, can lead to bowel cancer.

As with infections, we may need a helping hand from modern medication if cancer does start to take hold—antibiotics in the case of infections and surgery, chemotherapy or radiotherapy in the case of cancer.

Once we've had cancer treatment though, we need to look at our lifestyle with a view to keeping it away. If we needed strong antibiotics to treat food poisoning, and having recovered we started tucking into a plate of semi-raw fried chicken, people would think we were bonkers. And yet after cancer we often go back to our previous lifestyle and just rely on hope and prayer.

I'm certainly not saying that all cancer recurrences are preventable, or that if your cancer returns you are somehow to blame. There are many factors involved in the process of recurrence. However we can give ourselves the best chance. It may not be enough, but for some people it may make a difference.

Let me use an analogy. It's possible for any car to get stuck in mud. However, certain factors make it more or less likely. A Range Rover can get through quite deep mud unscathed. But if we own a rear wheel-drive Smart car, we probably shouldn't be tempted to take a short cut through a newly-ploughed field a few days after heavy rain. If we stick to proper roads though, we should be fine most of the time.

If the temptation to do a bit of off-roading in a Smart car became irresistible and we got stuck, we'd probably need the help of a local farmer and his tractor. Depending on how deeply we were entrenched, this may or may not work, and the car would probably suffer some collateral damage—a bent bumper or whatever. I don't think anyone would contemplate repeating the exercise on a regular basis.

So where I'm going with this?

Some of us are born with good genes or constitutions from a 'getting cancer' perspective (the top model Range Rover brigade). Some of us drew the Smart car straw – perfectly nice car, but not great in deep mud.

In the case of breast cancer, people who have certain genes—for example BRCA 1 and 2 could be thought of as Smart car drivers. You can't change your genes, and there are various other risk factors you can't do much about. Tall women have a slightly increased risk too (and stooping isn't going to help), as do women with denser breast tissue.

What you can do, though, is avoid the ploughed fields as much as possible—particularly if you have a Smart car predisposition to cancer. You shouldn't be complacent if you consider yourself a Range Rover either; there are some pretty deep ploughed fields out there, and some that haven't been mapped yet.

So let's look at the ploughed fields of breast cancer. First I want to tell you about the 'official' ploughed fields—the ones on the ordinance survey map of life.

The International Agency for Research on Cancer (IARC), and the World Cancer Research Fund together with the American Institute for Cancer Research (WCRF/AICR) have listed the factors, which have strong, researched evidence that they are associated with cancers. Depending on how much evidence is available, they are classified as 'definitely -associated' or, with slightly less evidence, 'probably -associated'. These are summarized below.

Definite Causes of Breast Cancer (proven correlation)

1. Alcohol: this raises sex hormones, but it's probably a general cancer promoter too. Risk increases with quantity, but even one unit daily has an impact, so it's quite serious. It's your choice, and life shouldn't be miserable. However, if you drink regularly you should have some alcohol-free days, and avoid drinking so much that you feel ill the next day.

2. The combined oestrogen/progesterone contraceptive pill: This is perhaps not surprising, as these hormones can stimulate some breast cancers. The good news is that if you stop the pill, your increased risk will have disappeared after ten years.

3. Combined hormone replacement therapy (HRT): for treating menopause symptoms. HRT contains the same hormones as the contraceptive pill. The increased risk disappears five years after stopping HRT. Oestrogen-only HRT carries less risk of breast cancer, but an increased risk of cancer of the uterus, so I'm afraid there's no quick win there.

4. Radiation: X-rays and natural radiation each account for 0.5% of breast cancers in women. This includes diagnostic X-rays (including mammograms) and radiotherapy. Between three and six women in every ten thousand who have regular mammograms will develop breast cancer as a result. So the risk is there—although small—and you must remember that mammograms may allow your cancer to be discovered earlier.

5. Body fat: this is a biggy, no pun intended (well, maybe). Having excess body fat is a strong risk factor in post-menopausal women, particularly stomach fat, especially if you've gained weight as an adult.

In pre-menopausal women the evidence is slightly confusing—the risk actually seems to be slightly lower in overweight women, at least in some ethnic groups. However (step away from that strawberry cheesecake) stomach fat may still increase risk, even in pre-menopausal women. The breast cancer rate was 79% higher in women with the greatest waist-to-height ratio compared with the lowest.

There's a logical reason why more body fat can predispose you to breast cancer. Once again it relates to female sex hormones, which are stored in fat tissue.

6. Breast feeding your babies *decreases* your risk of breast cancer, which is a bonus.

Probable Causes of Breast Cancer (slightly less evidence)

1. Night shift work: possibly because night-time light reduces melatonin levels, which leads to higher oestrogen levels.

2. Smoking tobacco: this increases sex hormone levels, in addition to being a known carcinogen.

3. A high fat intake: possibly due to associated obesity. However, there are good and bad fats, and some fats are both essential and beneficial in your diet—in moderation, of course.

4. Some medicines and occupational exposure to various chemicals. You should be warned if you are exposed to any of these.

5. Having fewer children and having your first baby later in life: both are associated with breast cancer, although this is unlikely to influence such life decisions.

6. Physical inactivity: Exercise probably protects against breast cancer, and of course may help with weight loss—so it's a double whammy.

This is the official list of definite and probable risk factors which we can influence—based on proven scientific data. However, there's information on other factors which can affect breast cancer risk—or any cancer, come to that. Some of these factors may never have sufficient scientific proof to satisfy the IARC and WCRF/AICR criteria, because studies are expensive and funding is limited.

This is where we need to use judgement. We can make educated guesses based on what seems rational, while at the same time dodging some of the crazier ideas. I'll share my educated guesses with you. I'm going to talk about nutrition, physical activity and mental/spiritual issues. All of these can affect your chances with cancer in my opinion.

First, let me tell you about David Servan-Schreiber. He was a French psychiatrist working in research in the USA when, in his early thirties, he was found to have a brain tumour. His outlook was considered very poor by his oncologist, who treated him with conventional anti-cancer treatment, but didn't expect him to survive.

Servan-Schreiber scoured the scientific literature for help in preventing his imminent death. He altered his lifestyle based on what he found, and has died just recently—some twenty years after his original diagnosis, and after a far longer life than expected.

His book talks about some interesting research and is a worthwhile read. I've drawn on some of his advice in this chapter.

So first let's see how nutrition and diet can help us. No, don't stop reading. I'm not planning to condemn you to a lifetime on some strict, miserable and boring diet, never again to chomp on a piece of gateau or enjoy a nice bottle of red. I am going to recommend ways in which you can still enjoy good food, but with the emphasis on *good*. The odd cream cake probably isn't going to kill you, but at least if you understand what foods you should be eating you can make better choices. And genuinely good food does actually taste good, and makes you feel better.

Nutrition and Diet

Cancer has become significantly more common over recent years in the west. According to Cancer Research UK, the incidence rates for all cancers in Great Britain have increased by over a third since the mid-1970s. 23% more men were diagnosed with cancer between 2009 and 2011 than between 1975 and 1977, and 43% more women. Having said that, this rapid rise seems to be slowing over recent years (it's still rising, but less quickly).

So why have western countries experienced such a dramatic increase? There are probably many reasons: more people are surviving to old age, when cancer is more common, for example.

However there is evidence that changes in our diet and lifestyle have played an important part too.

Another worthwhile read is The China Study, by T Colin Campbell—an American professor in nutritional biochemistry. He was a co-investigator in a large epidemiological study, looking at the relationship of diet to various illnesses, including cancer. The study was undertaken in China, because at the time Chinese communities had very stable populations and well-defined local lifestyles, and because there were well-documented disease statistics for these communities.

The China Study showed that rural Chinese communities consistently had a very low incidence of cancer and heart disease. They ate a mainly plant-based diet, using locally grown vegetables and cereals, and ate meat only on special occasions, such as New Year. They were very physically active, due to the nature of their work and lack of cars. Chinese office-workers in cities such as Shanghai had higher rates of those diseases, but still lower than in the west. Their diet, although still Chinese, had become slightly more western. They ate more meat, and they also had access to dairy foods, which are not traditionally eaten in China. They were less active than rural people, but as the bike was their main transport, they still did more exercise than their western counterparts.

The study concluded that a mainly plant-based diet with only occasional meat and an active life-style was the reason for the lower incidence of cancer.

You may think that maybe Chinese people just aren't predisposed to cancer, but other studies, such as those summarised by the USA National Cancer Institute, have shown that if people emigrate to the USA, from the second generation, their cancer risk rises towards that in their new country.

This would suggest that different life-styles are more important than their genetic make-up.

So how has our diet changed over recent decades in the west? As a child, I would pick vegetables and fruit with my mother in our allotment. We weren't unusual. It was a struggle for many people to feed their families. Our food was bought at local butchers and greengrocers and usually took the form of locally-sourced products, in season. We had little access to food from abroad—it was simply too expensive.

Convenience foods were unusual. They gradually became available during the middle years of my childhood, but even then they were relatively expensive. I remember my mother sharing a pack of two small beef burgers between the four of us. My father got a whole one, my mother had half, and my brother and I had a quarter each. A small block of ice-cream was called a family block, and treated as such. It was little bigger than a portion many people would finish off by themselves today. Similarly a 100g bar of chocolate was a family bar, and we each had a couple of squares maybe once a week. Economic necessity prevented most people from over-indulging. But now even people on low incomes can afford large quantities of cheap, processed foods. The difference now is not so much the quantity of food, but the quality.

Nowadays, we shop in massive supermarkets that offer exotic fruit and vegetables from around the world and fabulous arrays of delicious-sounding ready meals and deserts. But what about the nutritional quality?

Fruit and Vegetables
Fruit and vegetables are often transported, semi-ripe, around the world, and stored in refrigerators or in artificial atmospheres. They look beautiful, but have you ever noticed how different tomatoes and peaches taste if you buy them really fresh, such as in Italy or Spain? They actually have taste.

There are many arguments and counter-arguments regarding the nutritious value of mass-produced versus organic food, and of locally-grown versus shipped vegetables. Studies are cited for both sides of the argument and the data are inconclusive. However, logic would suggest that products picked naturally and eaten locally and which taste better probably are better.

Modern agricultural methods, aimed at increasing production and profit, mean that quick-growing vegetable varieties are often selected. There are fewer nutrients available in the soil than there were in the past, and much of the produce has less time to store nutrients such as vitamin C, because they are picked semi-ripe.

So the problem may be that not only do we eat less fresh fruit and vegetables than we used to, but in addition the quality may not be so good either. I can't tell you this is categorically true, but it is a concern of mine.

Meat, Fish and Dairy

Meat is much more universally accessible than it used to be. Chicken used to be an expensive luxury mainly enjoyed at Christmas. Now, with intensive farming, it is a cheap food. Other meats are also relatively cheaper than they were in the past, again due to modern farming techniques. Consequently many are eating more meat than previously.

Much of our fish nowadays is farmed, whereas it used to be predominantly wild-caught.

Does all this affect the quality? Well, we probably don't know the full implications of rearing animals in restricted conditions, and feeding them grain and special artificially formulated foods, but let's use omega-3 fatty acids as an example.

Omega-3 fatty acids are important in the cancer battle. If we have more omega-3s in our diet and less omega-6s, inflammation in our bodies is reduced. As I mentioned earlier, chronic inflammation favours cancer, so this is important.

The best source of omega-3 fats is oily fish. However, farmed fish are artificially fed, sometimes on grain and various other unnatural fish foods. Dependent on what they are fed on, the percentage of omega-3 fats can be less than in wild fish. The counter argument used is that farmed fish contain more fat overall, however I'm not convinced that needing to eat more fat for the same benefit is a great argument. The Washington State Department of Health have produced an interesting report covering this (see Further Information).

David Servan-Schreiber explains that grass contains omega-3 fatty acids, and spring grass is particularly rich in them. If cows are allowed to graze, instead of being kept in compounds and fed an artificial grain diet—as in some massive USA beef-producing establishments—their meat should contain more omega-3 too.

He also comments that free-range chickens, which forage for food, rather than only being fed a grain diet, produce eggs and meat with higher levels of omega-3 fatty acids.

These are examples where nature may know best. The differences in omega-3 content following different farming methods may or may not be important, but the long-term effects of our modern intensive farming methods may not be fully understood.

Although not proven, there is a concern that excessive meat consumption in modern-day western countries may be partly responsible for increased cancer rates.

Some protein in our diet is important and necessary for our health, and meat and fish is a good source of this. However, too much protein is not desirable. The body cannot store excess protein, so your liver has to work to break it down into waste products and carbohydrate. The carbohydrate will then be converted to body fat if it is surplus to immediate energy needs.

There are some theoretical concerns with milk and milk products too, and some people believe that dairy products are implicated in cancer, although this has by no means been categorically established.

Milk contains certain active agents which are useful for growing babies but may be associated with cancer in adults—for example Insulin-like Growth Factor-1 (IGF-1). This probably isn't a problem usually, and milk products such as cheese and yoghurt drinks are consumed regularly in India, a country with a relatively low incidence of cancer.

In the USA, however, cows are treated with IGF-1 to increase milk yield, which leads to increased IGF-1 levels in the milk itself (this practice is currently banned in Europe). It isn't proven that IGF-1 consumed in dairy products causes cancer, but it is certainly a concern, and another example where changing farming practices for commercial gain may have a sinister down-side.

Processed food
What about processed food, ready meals, 'low-fat' foods, high sugar deserts and sweets and so on? Nowadays they occupy a large portion of many supermarket trolleys.

There are many potential problems with these. Most processed foods induce a rapid rise in blood sugar. The body responds by producing insulin, which reduces this excess blood sugar by converting it to fat. However, this insulin spike lowers the blood sugar just a bit too much, making you feel hungry and causing you to crave more sugar. This vicious circle eventually leads to type II diabetes, heart disease and obesity. In addition several studies have shown an association between high blood sugars and cancer, particularly fatal cancer.

Convenience foods frequently contain trans fats too. Fats have been given a bit of a bad press over recent decades, but good fats are actually an important part of our diet, as we need the essential fatty acids (the clue is in the name) which they provide. Good fats may actually help us lose weight in several ways: by encouraging body fat break down, by making us feel full for longer and by slowing the release of carbohydrates into our blood.

However, trans fats are definitely not good for you. For a start, they're not natural; they've been manufactured for commercial reasons. You may see 'partially hydrogenated vegetable oil' on ingredient lists—these are trans fats, made by adding hydrogen to vegetable oil. They have a longer shelf-life than good quality oils, and are often used in deep fat fryers in take-aways. Whether trans fats affect cancer directly is currently unclear, however at least study (called E3N-EPIC) has shown an association with breast cancer and trans fat intake.

Processed foods not only contain trans fats and high proportions of fast-release sugars, but they contain little or none of the important micronutrients present in fresh vegetables. So if we are replacing fresh vegetables with ready-meals, we are depriving ourselves of important supplies for our immune system.

Processed foods fool your body too. Your body thinks it's eating a meat dish, for example, when in fact it contains high quantities of sugar or corn syrup. If we eat pure foods (simple meat, fish, vegetables and fruit) our body soon starts to tell us when we are really hungry, and what foods we need. We feel like eating carbohydrates when we need energy, and so forth. If we confuse our body by eating processed food, these clever feedback mechanisms fail to work, and our body starts to crave the wrong things. This is one reason why we put on weight.

A good example is artificially sweetened foods, such as diet drinks. The body tastes the sweetness and as it expects sugar, it starts producing insulin to mop up this sugar and turn it into fat. When the diet drink fails to deliver sugar, the insulin removes sugar from the blood anyway, lowering levels too much, which makes us hungry, so we eat more. This is probably why some studies, such as one by Fowler and colleagues in Texas, have shown that people who drink diet drinks actually put on weight.

Pro-inflammatory foods

As I mentioned earlier, cancers can harness aspects of inflammation to help them grow. Chronic inflammation also uses up valuable materials which our immune system needs to do its job. Certain foods promote inflammation and others suppress it, so it is useful to have the right balance in our diet. Examples of foods which promote inflammation are high sugar foods, refined carbohydrates, trans fats and red meat.

Foods which suppress inflammation include fresh fruit and vegetables, olive oil, flax oil, oily fish, whole grain foods and green tea. The observant amongst you will notice that these are the same foods which have already been discussed as harmful or beneficial with regard to cancer, so rather than involving yet more dietary rules, this just reinforces earlier advice.

Another important aspect of keeping inflammation under control is eating the correct balance of omega-3 and omega-6 fatty acids. Many foods contain these, and it is necessary to have both in our diet, but it is important to have more omega-3 than omega-6. It is the balance that matters. Oily fish and flax oil both contain high amounts of omega-3, and can can tilt the ratio in your favour.

Suppressing inflammation will also protect you from heart disease and inflammatory diseases such as rheumatoid arthritis.

So what should we eat?

I've listed some of the concerns, so how should we approach our diet in the face of them?

Well, in order to protect against cancer, the body's immune cells need a good supply of certain nutrients, much as an army cannot fight without adequate provisions. Many vegetables contain these necessary nutrients.

From all the available evidence, it would make sense to eat several different vegetables every day in order to feed our body gently and naturally with the numerous micronutrients we need to support our immune system. I would recommend trying to find locally grown fresh organic vegetables whenever possible, but if you can't obtain or afford these, you will still get benefit from any vegetables. The high colourings in some vegetables often indicate high levels of antioxidants, important for fighting cancer and infection, so choosing vegetables of varying colours has merit.

Fresh fruit is also good, but in moderation. Fruit contains fructose, which is a fast-release carbohydrate, causing rapid rises in blood sugar. It's good to include some fruit in your diet, but don't over-indulge, and always choose whole fruits, not fruit-juice, as the fibre slows absorption.

As with vegetables, eating a sensible amount of fish and meat, whatever the source, is probably fine but choosing organic/wild-caught and free-range options is preferable when you can. Consider using vegetable sources for proteins too, such as chick-peas and lentils for example. Encourage a low inflammatory environment by eating plenty of omega-3 fatty acids from oily fish, oils such as linseed (flaxseed) and rapeseed as well as nuts such as walnuts and pistachios.

If we have a varied and balanced diet of good quality fresh unprocessed food, we'll probably provide our body with sufficient nutrients on a daily basis to give our immune system the best support for surveillance and destruction of cancer cells. Daily consumption is important too because there are some foodstuffs, such as vitamins, which our bodies can't store or manufacture.

Some people advocate taking supplementary vitamins, as they don't believe modern food has the same goodness as it used to do; others say a good balanced diet is all we need. It's a personal decision. However, vitamin supplements are not a substitute for a good diet. Natural foods are designed to give you all the nutrients you need in suitable amounts. Some vitamin tablets are not well absorbed, and it would be difficult to take an array of pills to completely cover all the micronutrients we need to be healthy.

Some specific foods are worth a mention. Broccoli has hit the headlines recently because of its anti-cancer properties. Some pharmaceutical companies are attempting to extract these in order to concentrate their anti-cancer effect.

Turmeric also has natural anti-cancer properties. It's poorly absorbed from the gut, so pills simply containing turmeric extract are unlikely to be effective. However, taking black pepper and ginger with turmeric increases absorption, and as it happens, these ingredients are often eaten together in Indian cooking. My point here—and this is a recurring theme—is beware of cheating on nature and looking for quick wins. It's likely that various natural foodstuffs each contribute some nutrients which the body can use to fight cancer, and over thousands of years, cultures have developed the best ways to make use of them.

Soya is worth a specific mention with regard to breast cancer. Soya beans contain phytoestrogens, which are natural substances that mimic oestrogen. As we know, oestrogen can stimulate some breast cancers, therefore some people advise against eating soya products. However, phytoestrogens in soya compete with the body's own oestrogens, effectively blocking them. The soya oestrogen effect, in contrast, is much weaker. So there is another school of thought that soya actually protects against breast cancer. In countries where soya is a major part of the diet, breast cancer rates tend to be lower, which would add weight to this theory. The jury is currently out. Personally I do eat soya, and I believe that it does more good than harm.

There's a huge amount of useful information on good nutrition and cancer, and this is just a sprint through the current knowledge. You don't need a biochemistry degree, it's a matter of fairly simple choice. Go for 'proper' food, of the best quality you can afford. Eat lots of varied vegetables, slow release carbohydrates such as grains and sweet potatoes, eat oily fish and avoid excesses of meat and dairy. Avoid foods with a high sugar content such as sweets and desserts and avoid processed foods of any kind. Limit or (ideally) avoid alcohol and tobacco.

Physical Activity
The IARC list classifies lack of physical activity as having a probable link to breast cancer. There are some large-scale studies which support this, including a study of 25,000 women in Norway, by Thune and colleagues, which showed decreased breast cancer risk in women who did heavy manual labour or exercised for at least four hours per week. A study by Sheppard and colleagues in African American women showed similar benefits.

For health reasons it's very important to increase our activity level, at least to that for which our body was designed. Our activities for daily living involve much less exertion than they did a generation ago, due to labour-saving devices and cars, for example. This means that we need to make an effort to exert ourselves more in our leisure time and incorporate more activity into our life. Physical activity can also help with depression, which can often develop with cancer.

Which leads me conveniently to the subject of mental well-being.

Mental/Spiritual Wellbeing

There have been many debates on mental state and susceptibility to cancer. Not surprisingly, as our psyche is rather complex, studies have been inconclusive. It's difficult to tease out a single aspect of our mental state and study it in isolation.

As with diet, this isn't about attaching blame. Cancer patients didn't eat enough veg; they're needy wimps, and so on. This is absolutely not the case. Getting cancer is usually due to a combination of many factors. Nevertheless, it would be wrong to ignore the influence of the mind.

When we are stressed, our bodies produce various hormones, such as cortisol and adrenaline, which have numerous physical effects such as speeding our heart rate and raising blood pressure. Some studies have shown that they suppress elements of our immune system too. So it's theoretically possible for stress to inhibit our immunity to cancer cells.

Many people attribute cancer to a particular traumatic effect in their life, but this is always difficult to prove. People tend to look for a reason when bad things happen to them, and there's no way of confirming cause and effect. Maybe the cancer would have happened no matter what, and blaming a trauma is just post-hoc rationalization. This is true, but maybe a stressful situation *did* sometimes contribute; the fact is that we just don't have enough evidence to be sure at the moment. I have a couple of friends who developed aggressive cancer after serious work stress and bullying, and it's very tempting to believe that these events contributed to their illness.

We all suffer stress in our lives, and we can find ourselves in unhealthy situations in which we are physically affected by this. It wouldn't do any harm to address stress levels in your own life.

You may want to consider changing jobs, partners or friends if they are adversely affecting your mental health. In addition to general stress, a mental state of 'helplessness' seems particularly important. Once again, I would refer to Servan-Schreiber's book. He describes several fascinating studies. The first was in rats with cancer. They were divided into three groups. One group were fed and treated normally, and the other two groups were given short electric shocks—not harmful, but enough to be unpleasant—at random intervals. One of these two groups had no control over the shocks, but the other group had access to a lever and they learned that if they pressed this, the shock would stop.

Interestingly, in the rats which had no control over their shocks, more died of their cancer than in the other two groups. Their behaviour changed too. They became despondent, lost their appetite and their interest in sex.

However, the group who received the shocks but could control them with a lever survived their cancer significantly better than either of the other two groups—even the group who received no shocks at all, and their behaviour and eating patterns seemed unaffected by the shocks.

These were rats, not humans, but it does show how mental state can influence cancer resistance. Although it was a single small experiment, it indicates that helplessness can be more detrimental than just stress alone.

Servan-Schreiber describes other studies where higher-levels of inflammation-promoting agents were found in the blood of people feeling helpless, and we know that inflammation encourages cancer growth.

He also describes another study in Finland—this time in healthy young men. They were asked questions to assess whether they had significant feelings of helplessness. Six years later they were followed up. The number of men who had developed fatal cancer was 160% greater in the 'feeling helpless' group than in the other group, and three times more men had died in that group.

So if we are to reduce our risk of dying from cancer, it would seem sensible to work on our mental state. Many of us feel helpless for different reasons during our life—often relating to our experiences. For example helplessness in relationships, in the work situation and regarding our health. Sometimes we need help to overcome these feelings. It's well worthwhile seeking this help, which may be in the form of various types of counselling.

A situation that carries a huge potential to induce helplessness is cancer recurrence. We may have summoned up all our reserves to fight it the first time around. We may even have thought that we had beaten it. And then it comes back. We feel hopeless. We can't fight it again, it's going to get us in the end, we don't have the strength to go through all that treatment again, to tell everyone it's come back.

This is a situation in which support with dealing with these feelings of helplessness could have a real benefit to your outcome. You might not be able to overcome the cancer despite all efforts, but on the other hand, you may—and if not you may at least be able to extend and improve the quality of your survival. It really is worth a try.

In addition to counselling, and sometimes just the support of good family and friends, another powerful tool to optimize your mental state is meditation. What New Age kaftan-wearing thing is this, you may ask? Well actually, there's a growing body of evidence that you can use meditation to alter not just your mental state but your physical state too. The mind is far more powerful than we sometimes realize, and regular meditation has been shown to change various immune cells in a positive way, and to reduce inflammatory factors within our body.

Although one individual experience is not conclusive proof, the story of Ian Gawler makes compelling reading. He is an Australian vet, who developed a bone sarcoma (a particularly aggressive cancer) in his right leg at the age of twenty-five. He went through a number of conventional therapies but the cancer came back and he was given months to live.

In desperation he started meditating, for up to five hours a day at first, then he continued for three hours daily. Long story short, he is still alive forty years later, and has written several books on alternative ways to heal cancer. He also used various alternative treatments, including 'psychic surgery' and the Gerson diet (discussed elsewhere). Who knows what turned the tide for him, but he himself strongly believes that meditation was a major factor. It's easy to do, and it makes you feel better in many ways—so perhaps it's worth a try?

Sometimes getting cancer is a wake-up call. What are we accepting in our lives that are compromising our well-being and happiness? Maybe it's time for a spring-clean? Once again, I would recommend visiting a good counsellor. They explore with you whether you are attracting stressful situations or the company of stress-inducing people and what you can do to change this. You may be doing this by your behaviour, or your belief systems, which are based on your life experiences. Making your life happier and less stressful may help win the cancer war, and you'll certainly have more fun. Many people who get cancer do use this life-threatening experience to reconsider their lives, and a surprising number—myself included—eventually regard the cancer as a not you need the tractors of surgery and chemo- and radiotherapy to get you back on an even keel, to reduce the amount of cancer in your body to a level that the body's immune system can deal with. And sometimes, despite our best efforts and through nobody's fault, it just isn't enough. You may have individual factors which mean that your cancer gains the upper hand regardless of what you do, but I still believe it could help, and the advice is going to make you generally healthier anyway. Dr David Servan-Shreiber is an example of this; he did eventually die of his brain cancer, but enjoyed around 20 years more full and active life than doctors expected. Not such a bad outcome. Dr Ian Gawler is another example.

As stated earlier in this chapter, the *rate* at which cancer is increasing seems to be slowing down over recent years. However the actual numbers of sufferers is still rising, just less quickly, Cancer Research UK tells us that people born after 1960 now have over a 50% chance of getting cancer during their lives.

More people seem to be surviving cancer, though. Figures from the Cancer Research UK website in April 2014 show that survival from cancer has doubled over the last forty years in the UK. There are a few confounding factors here, as with everything else. Improved cancer screening programmes mean that many cancers are picked up early, and there is an argument that some of these may have been dealt with by the body and would never have come to light, thus inflating incidence and cure rate statistics. However it's hard to believe that this is responsible for all of these trends.

Possibly though, as people have become more aware of the dangers associated with fast foods and have started to revert to the healthier eating and physical activity levels of an earlier generation, the effects of this change are adding to the effects of better medical and surgical treatment.

Medical interventions continue to save many people who have developed cancer and are very important. However, the real answer for a happy, cancer-free drive through life, is to avoid ploughed fields in the first place by sensible driving. The oncological farmer's tractor really should be the last resort.

Summary:

Cancer cells constantly appear in our bodies. Maintaining a healthy immune system helps prevent these developing into full-blown cancer

Alcohol, 'The pill' and HRT are implicated in breast cancer

Therapeutic and diagnostic irradiation increase risk slightly

Excess body fat, smoking and high fat diet also increase risk

Aim to eat several fresh vegetables (ideally organic, locally produced, of mixed colours) every day

Eat some fruit but not to excess

Reduce chronic inflammation by increasing omega-3 and decreasing omega-6 fatty acids in diet

Avoid excess meat

Avoid all processed food

Aim to decrease mental stress

Try meditating regularly—it's easy and natural

Don't cheat on nature

Further Information:

'Anticancer: A New Way of Life' book by David Servan-Schreiber
The China Study by T. Colin Campbell, BenBella Books Inc
Dr Susan Love's Breast Book: S M Love with K Lindsey – Da Capo

Cancer Research UK	http://goo.gl/LwtWBC
Cancer Research UK	http://goo.gl/xcZXSi
National Cancer Institute	http://goo.gl/5aJMBv
Washington State Dept. of Health	http://goo.gl/gFkqwR
PLOS Medicine	http://goo.gl/w8dp9s
Breast Cancer Now	http://goo.gl/64zAAt
Cancer Research UK	http://goo.gl/yBThC3
Scientific American	http://goo.gl/4JAoI8
PubMed (NCBI)	http://goo.gl/dzkvdO
Science Daily	http://goo.gl/1voTDP
PubMed (NCBI)	http://goo.gl/U26ddz
Cancer Research UK	http://goo.gl/3T8XQT
PMC (NCBI)	http://goo.gl/GtSJH1
PubMed (NCBI)	http://goo.gl/6YS4QO
PubMed (NCBI)	http://goo.gl/lY6bxK
NHS Choices	http://bit.ly/1PSL5C2
PMC (NCBI)	http://goo.gl/oyVnjI
Cancer Research UK	http://goo.gl/SuwnhF
British Journal of Cancer	http://goo.gl/a4eisd
National Cancer Institute	http://goo.gl/Jw24Qi
Dr Ian Gawler	http://goo.gl/74Lm8K

Chapter 29

Meditations and visualisations which helped me

There are simple ways we can work on our whole system—mind, body and spirit. I will share a simple meditation that helped me while I waited for my surgery. You can use this, or adapt it to suit you. Anyone can do it. Sometimes you may sink into quite a deep state during the meditation. Sometimes your mind may be all over the place, and you may feel you have failed. Don't worry, there is no such thing as success or failure with meditation, it is what it is, and you will get out of the meditation whatever your being needs, even if you don't realise it, so just go with the flow. Try to do this regularly. Set aside a time of day when you won't be disturbed and can relax.

Sit in a supportive upright chair if possible, with your back resting against the back of the chair. Make sure your feet easily reach the ground, or rest them on a cushion (if you are unable to sit, just lie comfortably or whatever works for you). Make sure your mobile phone is on silent and that you won't be disturbed. Rest your arms gently on your knees.

Close your eyes and take deep slow breaths.

Ask God (or whatever you believe in) to protect you during your meditation.

Concentrate on your breathing.

If other thoughts come into your head, acknowledge them then let them go.

With your breathing, concentrate in turn on each part of your body, from your feet to your head, gradually letting each part—and all your muscles—relax.

Then visualise that you are sitting in a wind. You are being buffeted from all sides.

Imagine this wind is slowly becoming organised, starting to move in the same

240

direction, clockwise around your body, like a vortex.
Enjoy the feeling of calmness as the energy from the vortex strengthens and balances you.
When you are done, think about your breathing again.
Gradually wiggle your fingers and toes, and, when you are ready, slowly open your eyes.
Ask God to put a protective cover around you.
That's it.

You can do this for as long as you like; a few minutes is fine. If you enjoy the feeling, stay there longer. I think of Spiritual healing as a balancing of your body's energies too; you may have a different interpretation, depending on your religious or cultural beliefs. I have received spiritual and Reiki healing and found them very beneficial. I have given myself healing too. I'll share with you how I did this, in case you would like to try.

Sit as you would for the meditation above and concentrate on your breathing.
Imagine healing energies on your cancer.
When you are done, think about your breathing again and gradually bring yourself back to the present as in the previous exercise.
That's it.

When I used healing on myself, I thought of the cancer cells as cells that had gone off the rails, cells that needed guidance. It seemed to me that these cancer cells were part of my body, they were my cells, and it was better to treat them with love rather than as the enemy. Yes, they would eventually be removed during the operation, but in the meantime I intended to nurture all of my body, even the cancer cells.

My energies had been out of balance for a long time before the cancer was discovered. As with many people I'd had my share of emotional upsets. If I were to be cured, I believed that I needed to balance my energies as well as having the cancer removed. If I didn't treat my whole body, my mind and soul, the cancer could come back because I'd only treated the manifestation of the imbalance, not the root of it. These were my thoughts. We all have our own interpretation of our circumstances and what we need to do to deal with things.

241

Further Information:

Guided Meditations (Chopra)   http://goo.gl/nFVAgJ

Chapter 30

So let's recap

Well this has been a great deal to absorb—and I hope you've found it helpful.

Let's just go over the main points once more.

If you notice anything at all odd about your breast—not necessarily a lump—do consult your doctor, who should have a low threshold for referring you to a Breast Unit, where experts in breast disease, including cancer, work together to assess you and treat you if needed.

Nowadays almost everyone can expect good cosmetic results from breast surgery. There are many clever techniques to leave you with two normal-looking breasts, and you have every right to expect this, unless there is a good medical reason against it, in which case you should have this reason clearly explained to you.

You should fully understand everything that happens to you, and if you are feeling bewildered, stay glued to your seat across the desk from the doctor until you do understand. It's essential that you know what is being done to you and why, and what your options are, so that you can make the best decisions for your particular needs.

Your treatment will probably involve surgery plus or minus chemotherapy, plus or minus radiotherapy. You may need to take anti-oestrogen drugs afterwards. Exactly what treatment you need depends on the size of your tumour, what it looks like under the microscope and whether it has spread outside your breast.

The whole experience may take more out of you psychologically and physically than you realize for a long while afterwards, so be easy on yourself, and make sure you get enough rest.

totally negative experience.

My view of cancer treatment and prevention has changed. I used to believe that if you got cancer, the primary objective was to remove every last cancer cell from the body, and if you could achieve this, you'd be safe—cancer-free. But if you missed even a few cancer cells, they could hide away in the body, stealthily-growing, and when you least expected it they would come back and bite you in your oncological bottom.

There is an alternative way to look at cancer. We know that cancer cells appear in our bodies all the time, and the main reason we don't all get cancer is because most of the time our body successfully destroys these cells. Sometimes the body isn't able to destroy them and then cancer develops into a disease, as happens with infections.

Even if some cancer cells are left in the body after a cancer operation, the body is often able to find and destroy them (in some cancers more than in others). When cancer reappears after it's been removed, it's often due to the failure of these body's natural defences. Women who've had breast cancer have a slightly increased risk of getting a further breast cancer, usually in the opposite breast. This isn't thought to be a tumour which has spread from the original one, but a brand new cancer.

In her book, Dr Love talks about the phenomenon of tumour dormancy, where people seem to be cured of their cancer, then maybe ten years later they get a recurrence. So what puts the cancer to sleep and what wakes it up? Rather than worrying whether every last cancer cell has been removed, it may be more important to make sure the environment in your body doesn't favour cancer cell survival—either pre-existing cancer cells or new ones as they develop. This is where diet, physical activity and psychological health comes in. By providing your immune cells with a consistent supply of all the micronutrients it needs, you weight the odds in favour of your immune cells and against cancer. So eat good food as described earlier. Take steps to lower substances in your blood which may encourage the cancer cells— such as oestrogen in the case of breast cancer, various toxins such as alcohol and tobacco products and anything which increases inflammation. Finally, increase your level of physical activity and reduce your mental stress.

It seems to me that this is equally likely to benefit people who have incurable cancer. I'm not suggesting that by taking all these measures alone you will cure your cancer, and like the car stuck in the mud, sometimes

Most people survive breast cancer (two-thirds live at least beyond twenty years). Even if your cancer does come back, it is often possible to live with it—sometimes for a long time, sometimes not so long.

We all go through a grief process when faced with catastrophic life-events, including but not limited to terminal illness. The stages are denial, anger, bargaining, depression and acceptance. This is normal, and if we can work through to acceptance, we will find mental peace, even in the direst of situations. We may need professional help with this, both for ourselves and for people close to us who are going through it too.

NHS care is excellent, but sometimes for various reasons we don't get the attention we need, or we feel a mistake has been made. Try to learn as much as possible about your illness and the treatment, just as soon as you feel able. Request copies of hospital letters and keep them carefully.

Remember to speak out early if you are unhappy.

Respect yourself. Your attitude towards yourself can influence other people's attitudes. Be assertive, or people may overlook you.

If you feel your concerns are being ignored, try the following: ask to speak to someone senior; put your concern in writing; escalate to consultant, hospital CEO, PALS, as needed. You can also ask your GP to arrange a second opinion.

Demanding people tend to get attention. Make sure they are not stealing your share. But do remember that most healthcare personnel genuinely want to help, and don't forget that sometimes the doctor may be right. Be prepared to listen to their explanation.

Trainees need to learn, but if you don't want a trainee to attend to you, you have a right to say so.

There is a lot we can do to avoid cancer and reduce chances of a recurrence. Alcohol, birth control pills, HRT, obesity, smoking and high fat diets are known to be associated with breast cancer.

In general we need to maintain a healthy immune system through good nutrition, regular exercise and by reducing mental stress or removing any situation which leads to feelings of helplessness or lack of control.

Good nutrition means not overeating, eating fresh vegetables daily— ideally of different colours and locally-grown or organic if possible, eating some fruits but not to excess, eating only a moderate amount of meat and fish (preferably organic, free-range or wild-caught), eating foods containing omega-3 fatty acids regularly, avoiding processed foods, trans fats and sugar. Some foods have specific anti-cancer properties, such as broccoli and turmeric.

Exercise regularly and nurture your mental health. Take counselling if necessary and contemplate regular meditation.

Consider complimentary treatments to supplement your medical care—but not to replace it. There is a great deal of information on the internet, but there is no truth filter on Google, so beware of frauds or cranks. I have given you some tips on how to differentiate them from genuine research.

Finally, enjoy every moment of life, and don't miss opportunities to be happy. You never know what's ahead.

Lightning Source UK Ltd.
Milton Keynes UK
UKOW04f1807070116

266011UK00001B/2/P